Courageous

Caregiving

Courageous Caregiving

A High Calling

Lucy Dishongh

Bold Vision Books
PO Box 2011
Friendswood, Texas 77549

ISBN 9781946708007

Cover Art by Mirko Vitali / Dreamstime.com

Cover Design by Maddie Scott — ƙae Creative Solutions

Interior Design by ƙae Creative Solutions

Published in the United States of America

Dedication

To James, my forever love. Even in your dementia, you never forgot me, and you never let me forget that you loved me with all your heart. You were God's gift to me, to our children, and to all who were fortunate enough to know you.

To Matt, David, and Tim, my remarkable sons. Your are fantastic fathers, compassionate friends, and strong and godly men like your dad. Thank you for your love and concern for me since your dad's death. He would be very proud of you.

To Adam, Matthew, Micah, Brett, Jacob, and Savannah, my amazing grandchildren. You are my pride, my joy, and my constant inspiration to leave for you a legacy of faithfulness to God.

To Pam and Kathy. In my heart, you are my daughters, the grownup little girls I prayed for when my sons were little boys. I'm so grateful for your love and friendship. You are creative and talented, strong and industrious— true "Proverbs 31 Women."

To God, my faithful Guide and Friend. You have held my hand all my life, but much tighter during my thirteen-year journey as James' caregiver. You, who are the Author of life itself, have given me everything I have needed in order to finish this story—our story. I thank You every day for Your love and Your amazing grace.

A Special Thanks

To Ginger Couch, my sister in Christ:

You are one of the most loving, unselfish, gifted women I have ever known. My four hundred plus hand printed pages might never have become a "real" book had it not been for you. Over many months you miraculously deciphered my hand written pages. You typed and re-typed countless times as I edited and apologetically marked your beautifully typed pages with my ruthless red pen. Through it all, you never complained, and you were my greatest encourager. I call you my "one women cheering squad." I am so grateful for the priceless gift of your time, your skill, your love, the numerous ink cartridges, and who knows how many reams of copy paper.

"Ginger, *I will love you forever; I will like you for always.*"

To the Staff at Brookdale Pearland (formerly The Hampton):

Our home at The Hampton met all of our needs, providing rest, support, comfort, beauty, safety, and so much love. I will be forever indebted to all who lovingly served us there, providing things I desperately needed after caring for James for the first ten years of his illness. I have wonderful memories of our lovely, "custom-made" apartment, great friends and lots of thoughtfully and professionally planned activities. I especially treasure my memories of the last year of James' life which was spent in the secure and loving environment of Clare Bridge, Brookdale's highly acclaimed Memory-Care community. There his life was filled with meaning and purpose, and with people who skillfully cared for him, genuinely loved him and always treated him with dignity. He thrived and flourished there, touching the lives of all with whom he came in contact. I will always be grateful for the role Brookdale Pearland played in our lives during the last three years of our journey with Alzheimer's.

Table of Contents

FOREWORD

Don Piper

On how many occasions has it been my distinct privilege to unite a man and woman in holy matrimony? As I ask them to recite the wedding vows, I'm always mindful of the reality and utter significance of the promises they are pledging to keep as long as they both shall live. Most folks have heard the lines repeated enough that they can practically repeat them by heart. It's one thing to repeat them from memory and another altogether to faithfully practice them. Particularly daunting is the commitment to live together, "in sickness and health, to love and to cherish, until death do us part." No one who enters into holy matrimony can truly grasp the gravity of the vows that they are making at the moment that they make them. We humans keep making the vows anyway. And I keep leading men and women in those vows.

James and Lucy Dishongh exchanged their wedding vows in November 1957 and fervently kept them until he slipped the bonds of this life and began his new life free of Alzheimer's in September 2012. Like the hyphen on a tombstone, it's the time between those dates that matters. Lucy and James lived a magnificent love story that I predict you will come to celebrate through the pages of this important book, *Courageous Caregiving: A High Calling.* But this is not just the story of a married life well lived, it's a real-life saga of living out the especially demanding part of the wedding vows which specifically calls for supporting each other in "sickness."

For thirteen years Lucy and their extended family lived each day in the shadow of Alzheimer's disease that afflicted James. They didn't just survive however. The Dishongh family gave us a template for courage and forbearance, grace and triumph, love and hope. You are about to read that story and you will be uplifted.

God obviously foreknew that James would need a trained-nurse wife like Lucy to see him through the years of the steadily declining quality of life that Alzheimer's is. You'll find excellent insight into how a wife and extended family should care for a victim of this insidious disease often called, "The Long Goodbye." The book is filled with great resources that can help anyone coming to grips with caring for such an overwhelming commitment of care. But it's also a primer on how caregivers have to be sensitive about caring for themselves as well.

If it takes a village to raise a child, likewise it takes a village to get through the sometimes-excruciating health crisis that is Alzheimer's.

Lucy weaves her family account using poignant personal stories and lovely poetry, as well as excerpts from her personal journals recorded at the time of the actual events. So these events seem like they occurred just yesterday. Her personally transparent accounts will make you glad to have "known" the Dishonghs and their powerful and very personal journey of faith and yes, suffering.

In case you haven't gathered through my sharing I watched this family experience these challenges first hand, having known Lucy and James for several years, as well as having been a ministry colleague of Pam Dishongh at Pasadena Texas' First Baptist Church.

You'll admire and respect them all, too, as you read Lucy's "love letter" to James, *Courageous Caregiving: A High Calling.*

As the victim of a horrific accident myself, years of hospitalization, surgeries, and a lengthy convalescence I do know what it is to rely on others to care for your every need only to run the risk of neglecting their own needs. Lucy offers great insight into how to balance these necessities. And as the son of a mother who is currently residing in assisted living due to her own struggle with dementia I know firsthand the battles that families fight as they seek compassionate quality care for loved ones afflicted with diseases of the mind. In this book, Lucy has taught us all a lot about gracious, thoughtful, and loving care for sufferers of Alzheimer's and its like. With advancing lifespans here to stay, the growth of these sorts of illnesses will only increase. Lucy Dishongh is way ahead of the curve on how to approach such challenging health issues and she does it in the only way a wife who keeps her wedding vows can, "in sickness and health."

A deep sense of gratitude to you Lucy for your faith and fortitude!

Don Piper

New York Times Bestselling Author and Speaker

90 Minutes in Heaven: A True Story of Death and Life

Preface

"I urge you to live a life worthy of the calling you have received. Be completely humble and gentle; be patient, bearing with one another in love"
(Ephesians 4:1-2).

My "calling" began on my 65th birthday July 22, 1999, with two words, "It's Alzheimer's. This book began with my first journal entry the day before I heard those words from the mouth of James' neurologist. For the next thirteen years I journaled my feelings, experiences, and prayers. I discovered that journaling was a powerful way to deal with my fears and frustrations, proving to be very therapeutic, helping me to move forward as I honestly and unapologetically expressed to God what I was feeling.

Writing about my life as James' caregiver enabled me to see that even in the darkest, most painful seasons there were still moments of grace:

- James' delight in people
- His strong childlike faith and trust in God
- His wonderful, unique sense of humor which kept us all entertained
- His unwavering, unconditional love for me, for our children, and for everyone he met

Although our losses at times were beyond imagining, so were our unexpected gifts. Because he no longer had a past, James showed us how to live alongside him in the present, one day at a time.

In our culture, we often talk about Alzheimer's in the abstract, as a label, not in all its bittersweet concreteness. Now, however, because it is affecting so many lives, it has emerged from obscurity and is forcing us to acknowledge its stark reality.

During my caregiving years, I cared for James at home for ten years; at a Brookdale Personalized Assisted Living Community for two years; and finally at that same Brookdale's highly rated Alzheimer's and dementia care facility, Clare Bridge.

I discovered that what I was experiencing as James' caregiver was different from most of the memoirs I found which documented other caregiver's experiences. This is the reason I feel so passionate about telling my story. With God's help, perhaps I can bring a fresh, unique voice to this major public health problem, this epidemic, which is having and will continue to have a severe impact on millions of our aging populace and their families until a cure is found.

Dear fellow caregiver, whoever and wherever you are, it is to you that I owe the inspiration for this book you hold in your hands. Sometimes I will refer to you as "Beloved" – which means "priceless", "unique" and "noble." These words describe all devoted, courageous caregivers everywhere.

Five years ago after reading back over ten years of journal entries I decided it was time to share with others the things I had learned – lesson too valuable to keep to myself. As I began to write with the inspiration of the Holy Spirit, I realized that God is the Author and I am the character chosen to give flesh to this story of God's faithfulness during a time I could not have survived without His grace.

Through His Spirit, my faithful Father has walked with me every step of this writing process. It's a good thing because I soon discovered that writing is no "walk in the park." It's hard and challenging There were time I wanted to give up – like the time is September of 2015 when the whole manuscript was lost somewhere in "the cloud" never to be found. Thankfully the hard copy was still with us, and we survived that hurdle.

Beloved, it is my fervent prayer that my story will give you courage and bless you as you walk your own path. I also pray that when your journey is over you will look back over your caregiving years and see that Caregiving really is a High Calling.

Acknowledgments

Where to begin? There are so many people to whom I want to say, "Thank you." To our wonderful doctors, our church family, old friends, and our extended family members, whose love and concern have carried me through the past thirteen years, I say, "Thank you."

Micah, you patiently and lovingly taught your eighty-two-year-old grandmother to use a computer, something I've always wanted and needed to do. Thank you.

For thirteen years, I spent time each morning at my "Bethel," reading from God's Word and from favorite devotional books. I wrote what I was learning from others' experiences, insights and wisdom. I journaled thoughts, ideas, and quotes from many sources long since lost or filed away "somewhere." To every pastor, conference leader, teacher, and author whose insightful words have inspired me, I say, "Thank you."

In the preface of his book, *Angels: God's Secrets Agents*, Billy Graham writes, "To everyone whose books and article I have read, I express my gratitude."[1]

I love what Karen Porter said in the acknowledgments of her delightful book, *I'll Bring the Chocolate:* "If you see something in this book that originated with you, please know that the use of it without your name is a mistake of the head, not the heart."[2]

Along with Dr. Graham and Karen Porter I say, "If you see any thoughts expressed in this book and they sound a little too much like yours, please forgive me.'"

I must acknowledge a special author and friend, Don Piper. Along with Cecil Murphy he wrote his extraordinary story, *Ninety Minutes in Heaven*, which was published in 2004. While serving alongside Don at

1   Billy Graham. *Angels: God's Secret Agents,* (Thomas Nelson Inc.), 2000.

2   Karen Porter. *I'll Bring the Chocolate, (Multnomah Books) 2007.*

my church, where he was serving on the ministerial staff, I discovered that he is an amazing man. Although he was still struggling with ongoing health problems from his accident, he was full of joy and zest for life. He encouraged me as I dealt with James' progressive dementia. I knew that during this time Don was writing his story. In the fall of 2008 Don said to me, "Lucy, write your own story about your life as caregiver to James. There are millions of caregivers just like you who will need your powerful message of God's faithfulness in times of adversity. I know you can do it." My book is the result of his encouragement and belief in me. Thank you, Don.

I've always believed that God works in mysterious and amazing ways. That was made clear the night I met Karen and George Porter. I had just finished my book, but I had no idea what to do with it. I was attending a Bold and Beautiful women's event at Grace Church Houston, and I was intrigued by a workshop which offered suggestions and helps for would-be writers. Outside the door to that conference, I met a charming woman and her husband. The Porters told me about their publishing company, Bold Vision Books. Thus began this "journey" together.

Karen, I still have to pinch myself when I think of the way you have blessed me with your belief in me and my story. Thank you.

Introduction

One Life Made Up Of Many Stories, One Story at a Time

Beloved Caregiver, no one else can tell our story for us. I'm telling mine. Tell yours.

Our story is made up of many stories from the past, the present, and the future. It is essential that, as caregivers, we remember and tell the whole story about the life we have shared with the person to whom we are now giving care. The "rest of our shared story" explains why we are faithfully, lovingly, and tirelessly serving beside our loved one with Alzheimer's disease.

Ours is a narrative that includes moments of breathtaking joy, gratifying companionship, and (for spouses), blissful romance before the intrusion of Alzheimer's forever changed our story. Our memorable experiences remind us why we now embrace with love and devotion the role and responsibilities of caregiving.

Our narrative is also a storehouse of treasures; a rich resource. It reminds us that this disruptive season of Alzheimer's is only one small part of a wonderful, full life we have shared with our loved one. It reminds us that this is not all there is. It also reminds us of how we came together and how and why our lives are still being woven into a tapestry of love.

The memories of the "rest of our shared story" are what sustain us in this heartbreaking time of indescribable sadness, this season where Alzheimer's is our constant companion. These memories can:

> lift our spirits,
>
> quiet our fears,
>
> ease our stress,

make us smile and laugh,

comfort our broken heart.

The "rest of our story" can lead us to proclaim to God and to all who hear our story, that we are thankful for all our days and years together, including this difficult, disruptive season. It can also remind us that we are who we are because of the fullness, significance and completeness our loved one brings to our life.[3]

In 1999, two words, "It's Alzheimer's", brutally and relentlessly rewrote the script James and I had envisioned for the next thirteen years of our life. From that gut-wrenching moment on, everything changed. The changes came slowly at first. Then finally, the threat to our dreams could no longer be denied. It soon became apparent that the future we had planned and dreamed of was now and forever beyond our grasp.

Slowly, but surely, over the course of the next four years, I became the mother, and James became my "little man." I think, for me, this role-reversal has been the hardest part of this disease to accept. I had always been James' "Princess." He had always been my "knight in shining armor." It was not that I was spoiled, weak, or helpless. I was extremely independent, but James loved his role as my protector, my champion. He had also been the spiritual head of our family. Now this terrible disease was robbing both of us of the way we had defined ourselves in our relationship and our marriage. As my tasks as caregiver to James became more demanding, more physically exhausting, I found that my role was becoming as much the "loving caregiver" as the wife and loving partner to James.

Once, in 2004, when I was helping James dry off after his shower, he looked at me and said, "Am I your little boy?" I replied, "No, you're my husband." To which he replied, "Boy, am I lucky." There were times when his "window" of perception opened, and he would say, "I'm a nothing and a nobody. I can't remember anything. My "memory button" is broken. Do you think we can fix it?" Then, for a brief time, he would seem depressed and troubled. I always reassured him that I loved him

---

3   Thoughts and excerpts from a Plenary given at a Caregiver's Conference and from a paper by Earl E. Shelp, Ph.D., Interfaith CarePartners Conference, Houston, Texas.

and needed him as much as ever. I told him that he was, and always would be, extremely important to me and our children.

There were times in the early years of our journey that I felt my life was "spinning out of control." I often felt 'fragile' and alone. Although I wondered at times if anyone knew what I was experiencing, in my heart I always knew that God did. He was with me, and he knew and understood. From the first day of this journey, I have turned to God, my source of strength, hope, and comfort.

One day, at my "Bethel," God showed me a verse, Deuteronomy 30:20. "Now choose life… that you may love the Lord, your God, listen to His voice and hold fast to Him. For the Lord is your life." With this promise and assurance, I began to "hold fast" to Him, to cling to Him daily in my desperation. Without fail, I found in Him all that I needed for each day. I learned to live one day at a time, not worrying about tomorrow. Along with my faith in God, it was my memories of the love James and I shared that sustained me. They were my lifeline to the past, my key to surviving the present, and my hope for the future.

I realize now that those thirteen years were only a small part of the beautiful life James and I shared. Those years, even though difficult, were not all that we had.

Beloved, in our sad moments,

our despairing moments,

our exhausted moments,

our seemingly hopeless moments,

we must remember the "rest of our story."

Then we will be comforted by all the things that gave us joy, all the times when our hearts overflowed with love and gratitude for the blessings of being with our loved one.

Our memories cannot change what is happening now, but they can give us the strength to meet the next challenge on our path. I keep a small picture of James on my bedside table, a picture taken our first Christmas together. It shows the face of my incredibly handsome young husband, still the love of my life. When I look at the pictures of us together on our honeymoon, vacations, at holidays, with our sons and grandsons, I remember vividly the events and experiences that gave us so much joy.

James, an avid photographer, took hundreds of pictures through the years with his wonderful Kodak Retina camera. After developing Alzheimer's, he could no longer remember how to use it. I keep it safely stored away, and I often look at it and remember those years.

I believe that God allows joy and sorrow to co-exist in our lives as part of the human condition in an imperfect world. I will surrender to God my Comforter, the sorrow, and I will embrace the joy. Even in our darkest valley, we can be sure that God is walking with us. He understands our sorrow and frustrations. He tells us to be at peace, to appreciate beauty and simple pleasures, and to depend wholly on His grace that is always more than enough.

We are tempted to ask in the midst of our heartache: "Where is the beauty of a mind that is void of memory and reasoning and logic? Where is the beauty of an existence where bodily functions fail and make one dependent on others for their basic needs? Where is the beauty when the 'Good-bye' to our loved one lasts for years?"

For some questions, there are no answers. We can, however, respond with love and patience to the weakness, dependency and loss our loved one is experiencing. With God's help and our love, we can find new and unique ways to cherish, enjoy, and find fulfillment with our loved one during our caregiving season. Some of my most precious memories of James are from the last two years of his life. Just snuggling with him on a small love seat at Clare Bridge, holding hands, watching him respond with so much humor and love to those who came and went —care associates, the family members of other residents, and visitors. I loved watching their faces when he asked, "Have you always been that pretty" or "that wonderful?"

Yes, Beloved, the storms are real,

the winds of discouragement are strong,

the lack of sleep is draining,

the drudgery is almost unbearable,

the changes are frightening,

the future is dark and uncertain,

the loneliness and loss are devastating.

But we are never alone. Jesus walks beside us, taking upon Himself our pain, our heartache, our disappointments, our fears. He wants to bless us today and comfort us in all our tomorrows. As our Burden-Bearer, He will carry our load when we are too tired to carry it further. In addition to this, He will provide new experiences that will enrich our lives and give us strength for today and hope for tomorrow. With His help we will not only be survivors, we will be overcomers.

PART ONE

Memories: The Rest of Our Shared Story

Chapter 1

A Walk To Remember When Life Unravels

When you meet that "perfect" someone,
But you lack courage to love without fear,
Go ahead. Love as if it's never going to hurt,
Because the Creator of love will always be near.
~Lucy

It's Father's Day, 2012. James and I are holding hands and cuddling on our love seat at Clare Bridge. James has lived in this wonderful Memory Care facility at The Hampton at Pearland, Texas for the past eight months. We have just finished breakfast, a special Father's Day event called "Let's Tie One On." All six of the men residents are sporting neckties. James, with his beautiful blue eyes, is wearing a blue shirt and tie.

I say to him, "Honey, you look incredibly handsome today." James looks at me adoringly and says, "You're too wonderful to be real. I've only known you for a few hours, but I love you with all my heart."

His words were totally unexpected. But I quickly recovered, and I said, "I love you, too, with all my heart. Do you want to marry me?" James got so excited, and with a huge smile he said, "I'd be crazy not to. Do you think we can?"

It was a bittersweet moment; a startling Deja Vu moment. I was back in a little park in College Station, Texas, fifty-five years ago, saying the same words: "Do you want to marry me?" James was responding with almost the same words: "Of course I do. I'd be crazy not to. I love you with all my heart. Will you marry me?"

꿍

This incident on that memorable day in 2012, James' last Father's Day, both thrilled and broke my heart. The memory of that day will be with me as long as I live. I've wanted so much during these last few years for James to remember even one small detail, one brief moment of our courtship and wedding. I wanted him to be able to share with me even one little memory from that special time in our lives. At the same time, I am so grateful that there is one thing he has never forgotten: he loves me "with all his heart."

It has been over thirteen years since James and I embarked on this journey into uncharted territory. It was a journey into the darkness and unknowns of Alzheimer's disease. It was also a journey filled with wonderful memories of a full, rich life of two people brought together by a loving, gracious God.

I've never been a risk taker. I prefer to stay on a well-marked trail, accompanied by a trusted guide and good friends. I like day travel with the sun lighting the path. This may explain why I never went on blind dates. It was a rule I firmly adhered to while I was a student nurse. However, one day in a moment of weakness, I agreed to go to a football game with the friend of my good friend, Arnold. Only God could have orchestrated that first date with James.

When I met James on that "improbable" blind date in October of 1956, one of the first things that attracted me to him, other than that he was gorgeous, was his quiet, calm spirit. I first interpreted this as shyness, but I later realized it was peace and contentment. He had a deep faith and wisdom rooted and grounded in God. Small talk was not easy for him, but, as his friends have expressed many times, when he spoke, you listened. I soon learned that his strength lay in the fact that he knew who he was, or I should say, "Whose he was." He loved the Bible, and his favorite verse was Proverbs 3:5-6: "Trust in the Lord with all your heart and lean not on your own understanding. In all your ways acknowledge

Him and He will make your paths straight." *The Message* translates the last part: "will keep you on track."

James was on track. He was, by far, the godliest man I had ever met. After fifty-five years of marriage to him, I can still say this with complete honesty.

⁊⁊

As I spent more time with James, I experienced his strength, his joy, his integrity, his sense of humor, his faith. I felt in my heart that I could trust him with my future. I had fallen in love with him from the beginning. I've always said that I fell in love with his reflection in a mirror, a story I tell later in "A Stroll Down Memory Lane."

Love, however, is more than just a word. It's the embedding of your life and all your future days and years with that of another person. It's trusting everything you are and hope to be to that person who, whether you acknowledge it or not, is at first a stranger, an uncharted path, an untested guide. It's a lifetime commitment to face together, with that one special person, whatever life will bring. It's sharing each joy and sorrow, even possible suffering or dementia, and eventually, death.

This is the kind of love I had always dreamed of for myself. I have seen it lived out in the lives of my parents who were completely devoted to one another. It's the kind of love I saw beautifully demonstrated about a month before my wedding to James.

As a Registered Nurse, I was doing vacation relief for several friends who worked in doctors' offices in Houston. I was busy planning my wedding and had not yet taken a permanent position anywhere. This particular day I was working in the office of one of my favorite doctors. At about 8:00 A.M., an elderly lady walked in to have her blood pressure checked. She was on a new medication and needed to be checked every week for the first month.

I could tell that she was in a hurry so, although she did not have an appointment, I took her blood pressure. As we talked, she shared that she had an appointment at 9:00 A.M. I asked if she had a doctor's appointment, and she said, "No. I need to go to the Nursing Home to eat breakfast with my husband." She told me that he lived there because he was a victim of dementia. I asked if he would be worried if she were a little late. She said, "Oh, no. He hasn't known who I am for the past two years."

I was surprised and I asked her, "You mean you still go every morning even though he doesn't know who you are?" She looked at me kindly and said, "He doesn't know who I am, but I still know who he is." As she left I couldn't hold back the tears. I thought, "This is the kind of love I want for my marriage. This is the kind of wife I want to be for James."

Sometimes I go back into my memory bank to reflect on this story. I know now that true love is not just physical or romantic. I know that true love is an acknowledgment and acceptance of all that has been, will be, or will not be. Is it a coincidence that I remember this story so vividly? Was it a coincidence that God allowed me to experience this profound lesson in love and devotion? I don't think so. I believe that He was preparing me, even then, for what lay ahead for James and me forty-two years later.

The last few days before our wedding I was very busy, as most brides-to-be are. I was so excited, and I was enjoying every moment of the preparation for the day I had dreamed of all my life. November 8. 1957, on the eve of our wedding, however, I had a case of pre-wedding jitters.

James and I were on our way back to my apartment after the Rehearsal Dinner. I remember the scene as if it were happening yesterday.

I said to James, "Honey, are you nervous about tomorrow? I love you so much, but I must admit – I'm scared. During the rehearsal, the finality and reality of this suddenly hit me. You know that I love you with all my heart, but I realize that I don't know you. Tomorrow I'll be placing my entire life – my future, my hopes, my dreams in your hands for the rest of my life."

James was quiet until we pulled up in front of the apartment. He may have been thinking, "What am I getting myself into?" Then again probably not, knowing James as I do now. Knowing him, I also realize just how hard it was for him to "bare" his heart so freely and beautifully to me that evening. Putting his arms around me, he said, "I'm scared too. But I love you so much. I don't want to spend another day of my life without you. We can't know the future, but we can trust the One who holds our future." He continued with one of the most moving sermons I have ever heard: He said, "I believe and trust that, before either of us was born, God planned for us to build a life together, starting tomorrow. He knows the plans He has for us to serve Him together to make a difference in our world. I promise you that with His help I will love you and take care of you for as long as I live."

By now tears were running down my cheeks. I thanked James for his beautiful words. Then I prayed a prayer thanking God for this wonderful man He had placed in my life. I prayed for God's peace for that night and for His blessings on the home we would begin the next day. I also prayed that He would protect us from anything that the 'enemy' might use to try to destroy the love we shared and the home we would build together. In that sweet moment of surrender of my fears to God, I found peace and courage. I found the confidence I needed for our future and the freedom and joy to love without fear of the unknown. I wouldn't trade the memory of that night for anything. Never again, since that night, have I doubted God's purpose in leading us together. I realized then, as I do now, that with God's guidance we could face anything that the future might hold. I was equipped and ready to risk the incredible journey He had planned for us.

Looking back, I can see how God began that night to weave our lives into a beautiful tapestry of love – His love for us and our love for one another. It is a love that continues today, unchanged by aging, the thirteen years of the dementia of Alzheimer's, and the inevitable reality of death.

I will refer to James in the next chapter as perfect. Was he? No. Our life together was not perfect. But it was continually being woven into that beautiful tapestry of love born out of our faith in a Perfect God and Father. It was a love that endured the unendurable and was sustained even when, with one word, "Alzheimer's," life as we knew it began to unravel. On that day, July 22, 1999, God, our faithful Guide, was there ahead of us, supporting us with His strength.

"And we continue to shout our praise,

even when hemmed in with troubles."

Romans 5:3 (*The Message*)

Our story is a rich, full account of two people who were in love for over fifty years—and thousands like us—for whom forever vows suddenly and terrifyingly have an expiration date. None of us wish to experience the slow, insidious theft of our loved one by Alzheimer's disease, but, unfortunately, many of us will.

I believe that God has chosen me to share our story with all of you who, with your loved one, are walking the valley of Alzheimer's. Your journey has been on my mind since I began writing this documentary of our journey. In fact, you are the primary reason I am remembering and 'reliving' our story, as painful as it has been at times.

My goal and purpose is to share with whoever may need it the strength, endurance, courage, and wisdom I discovered as caregiver to my most precious possession – my husband, James. I can assure you, from experience, that with God beside you, you will never walk alone.

My story is a love story, as you have probably figured out by now. It's a story not only about finding the love of my life, but also of losing him, slowly but steadily, to the ravages of Alzheimer's disease. I believe that God wants me to remind you that love is the thread that holds us together on this difficult path; this detour that was not in our original plans. However, I believe it is a part of God's permissive will. He knew that Alzheimer's would be a huge obstacle on our safe, predictable path through life with our loved one. Nothing startles God or takes Him by surprise. He has loved us, prepared us, and equipped us for such a time as this, even before we were born. He wants us to tap into His unlimited resources as we regroup and prepare to face the unknowns ahead. Trust me, you will need all the help He will give you because love's greatest trials are ahead on your journey with Alzheimer's.

There may be days when you want to give up and run away to escape the disappointments, the drudgery, the discouragement, the fears, the sadness. We caregivers all have days like that. I found that the best solution for those times was to go to my quiet place, my "Bethel", and spend time with God, talking to Him like the Friend that He is, pouring out everything that I was feeling.

I hope that you, too, will find your quiet place, your "Bethel." While there, listening to God speak through the Psalms or other favorite Bible passages, we will find ourselves experiencing the peace and comfort that only He can give. We can find courage in the truth that He is always with us, aware of our particular need at that very moment. Sometimes I was so desperate, I almost ran to my Bethel. I was never disappointed. God met me there, held me with His love, and rewarded my trust with His comfort, encouragement, strength, and renewed energy and resolve.

God wants me to share with you a great truth from His Word, one with which you may already be familiar: "Who shall separate us from the love of Christ? Shall trouble or hardship or persecution or famine or nakedness or danger or sword? No, in all these things we are more than conquerors through Him who loved us" (Romans 8:35, 37). With God's help, we will be conquerors and overcomers.

For my journey, I chose God's wonderful gifts known as the fruit of the Holy Spirit (Galatians 5:22). These are things you will need to successfully navigate the minefields of Alzheimer's: love, joy, peace, patience, kindness, goodness, faithfulness, gentleness, and self control. Hopefully, you will choose them.

So, beloved fellow traveler, put on your walking shoes and come with me as I share with you "Memories: The Rest of Our Story" and the continuing story, "Our Journey Into The Unknown of Alzheimer's." I sincerely hope I will prove to be a faithful guide. I received my training from the Master Guide. He is Almighty God, who goes before us and who knows every path, every valley, every mountain because He created them.

I must warn you…

there will be rivers to cross,

valleys to walk through,

obstacles, roadblocks, and detours to endure,

seasons to pass through,

storms to survive,

difficult decisions to be made.

But we will never be alone. God will be walking ahead of us, beside us, and behind us every step of the way.

I am so honored that you, wonderful reader, would trust me with your time, your heart, your pain, your fears, your hopes while on your own journey. Our backpacks are already filled with every provision we could possibly need for this journey. These provisions are all generously supplied from the storehouse of our Heavenly Father, our Guide, who has an endless supply of everything. We will only have to ask, and our needs will be met – at exactly the right time.

Many of the provisions in our pack are things that, for years, you may have taken for granted. Perhaps you have never even thought about them being from God, but they are extremely important for a successful journey: this journey through unfamiliar, uncharted, often hostile territory.

We may feel like trailblazers and, in a sense, we are. However, we only need to look in the Bible to find that others before us have embarked on their faith journeys. Men like Moses, Abraham, and Jacob, to name a few, have left familiar, comfortable lives to follow God in obedience. They, too, have journeyed to strange, unfamiliar, often hostile lands, with only their faith in God to lead them. Their success stories have encouraged me to share my story with those who will follow behind me. I want to continue my legacy of faith passed down to me from my grandmother and my parents. It is a legacy that each generation is responsible to pass on to the next.

My prayer is that all who will follow behind me will find me steadfast and that God will be glorified by my faithfulness and obedience. I also pray that my transparency and vulnerability in sharing my story, my memories, will bring significance to the characters and events of the story. My goal is that my documentation will encourage others and will create a moving, meaningful experience for all who will read it: my family, my friends, and all the countless, beloved caregivers who have started or will someday be starting their own journey with Alzheimer's disease.

Chapter 2

A Stroll Down Memory Lane

So many memories flood my mind
Of days so precious, left behind.
Memories, some fresh, some just a blur
Of who we are, who we were.
~Lucy

This is my story. Actually, it's God's story, one He has allowed me to be a part of; a story He wants me to share with you. Let me warn you men: it's a "chick flick." After all, it's a love story. One that begins with the classic opening words, "Once upon a time."

I've always been a dreamer. I guess you could say that I've always looked at life through rose-colored glasses. I'm also a hopeless romantic. I fell "in love" with every boy I dated, and I fell "out of love" as easily. I know that my righteous father and mother often prayed for a nice, stable, "grounded" man to come my way and stop my ceaseless, butterfly dance through life. As promised, God always answers "the powerful, effective prayer of a righteous man" (James 5:16b).

My parents' prayers were answered one day in October of 1956. I was a student nurse in my senior year at Lillie Jolly School of Nursing in Houston, Texas. One day, in a whimsical moment, I agreed to a blind date to the University of Houston – Texas A&M football game. My date was the friend of a mutual friend, Arnold. He told me that his friend was one of the best men he had ever known. I never went on blind dates, but I had just broken up with my "mission volunteer" Aggie, and I was feeling vulnerable. Of course, looking back, I know that God was in all of the details that October day.

When I stepped off the elevator in the Student Nurses Residence where I lived, I saw a perfect man reflected in the full-length mirror across from the elevator doors. I saw black wavy hair; eyes so blue I could see them across the large lobby; a beautiful smile; perfect teeth; clothes tailored to fit his trim body perfectly. I was in love. I never imagined that this perfect man was my date. I wanted him to be. Then I saw Arnold standing beside him, and I knew.

I didn't know then, but I know now that God orchestrated that whole situation for me as part of His plan for my life. I always said later, as in the song from the *Sound of Music*, – "somewhere in my youth or childhood, I must have done something good."

Arnold introduced this perfect man, James Dishongh (beautiful man, beautiful name). I can tell you now as I could have then, he was not in my plans. I had already decided that God had called me to be a Missionary Nurse in Africa. Two years before, I had left my Pre-Med studies to enroll in Nurses' School. I seldom ever dated anyone who was not a Mission Volunteer or a Ministerial student. I was very focused.

That first date was fun and stress-free, except when James yelled, "Come on, Big Red"—while my heart was on the field with my beloved Aggies. I felt like punching him in the nose at times, but I didn't want to damage his perfect face. My father was on the faculty at Texas A&M, and I was an Aggie through and through. I let it be known that I had season tickets to all the Aggie home games at Kyle Field.

The day after our first date, James called to see if I still had tickets to the sold-out Homecoming game between Texas Tech and Texas A&M the next weekend in College Station. With a touch of arrogance, I said, "Yes." He said, "I thought maybe you could use one, and I could use one, and we could go to the game together." And that is how our second date occurred – the date on which we felt something special happening between us.

That Saturday, game day, James drove us to College Station. We had lunch with my parents and my sister. My father made his famous chili-cheese hot dogs. My parents and my twelve-year-old sister fell in love with James that day. James with the beautiful blue eyes, the beautiful smile, the beautiful heart. I think my parents sensed that day that God was preparing to answer their prayers for my future.

I've always heard that God works in mysterious ways. As improbable as it seemed, a tornado hit Kyle Field during the game, and James and I were forced to go below the stands. James took off his jacket, put it around me and held me until the storm subsided. He was so protective and attentive. I felt strangely nurtured by this amazing man. Because everything was wet and covered by debris, James and I left the stadium and listened to the rest of the game from the safety of his car at Stuart's Drive-In in College Station. We talked for hours about everything.

When James took me home, as a spectacular moon rose in a beautiful clear sky, he kissed me. (I can still remember that kiss.) The sweetness of the day and of that moment overwhelmed me. I knew I had never felt that way before.

After James had left to go to his home in Bedias, I felt as if a part of me was missing. I didn't want to feel that way. Remember, I had big plans for my future. For the next six months, I avoided James' calls, but I never forgot him.

In April, 1957, I answered the phone by my room in the dorm. It was James' dear voice. I was defenseless. I had no ready excuse for him or myself. We went to see the movie *Funny Face* at the Alabama Theater. James held my hand and, although he didn't kiss me, there was that "something special" between us. As I signed in, the night Housemother winked at me. I must have been glowing. I could tell that she approved of James. Who wouldn't? He was quiet, polite, and—did I mention?—perfect.

Several weeks passed, and though we talked on the phone occasionally, we did not see one another. The Senior Student Nurse picnic was coming in May, and I became obsessed with the idea of taking James as my date. I tried calling his apartment. No answer. I finally reached his sister, Marie, who told me that their father had suffered a stroke. James had been driving back and forth from his job with Shell Oil Company in Houston to Bedias every evening to check on his father. I know now that was typical behavior for James, the most caring, unselfish person I've ever known. I realized that, although I barely knew him, I respected him and admired him. Somehow, I wanted him in my life.

Marie promised to get in touch with James and have him call me, which he did – that same day. He said that he would very much like to take me to the picnic. In *The Message,* Eugene Peterson's paraphrase of *Jude* 2 is wonderful: "Open your hearts, love is on the way." I decided that, with God's help, I would be submissive to whatever He had planned for me.

The day of the picnic was beautiful. The magic had begun. I remember every detail of that day in May of 1957—every perfect moment. I felt like a princess. I didn't wait for the desk to send for me. I signed out and waited for James. Remember, this was only our fourth date. When I saw him, my heart pounded; he was even more handsome than I remembered. He took my hand and led me to a beautiful new car, a black and white 1957 Ford Fairlane 500 with a Thunderbird engine. I said, "This is a different car, isn't it?" And James said, "Yes, I bought it for you." I told you this is a love story.

James drove me home to College Station that evening after a wonderful fun-filled day. I sat very close to him, and my heart sang all the way home. After that day, James and I began seeing each other as often as possible with his job and my very busy schedule of trying to finish school and graduate. Sometimes we went to a movie or out to Hermann Park to walk around the lake.

One night we went to the Metropolitan Theater to see one of the "Tammy" movies. The theme song was *Tammy's in Love.* On the way back to the dorm, this song was played on the radio. At the end of the song, I turned to James and said, "I love you." Thankfully, we were in front of the dorm by then because, otherwise, we might have wrecked. The reality of what I had just unexpectedly said hit both of us. It was several days later, out at Hermann Park, that James said, "I love you, too." Because he never spoke lightly or frivolously, I knew he meant it.

I had been offered a job as Head Nurse of the College Infirmary at Texas A&M starting the first of July, right after graduation. I decided to accept the offer. I felt that I needed to go home and spend time with my family. I also wanted time to think and pray about my future.

James and I cried the night before I left, but we both knew that mine was a wise decision. For the next few weeks, I prayed earnestly for direction. With a new found submission, I surrendered my plans to God's greater plan, and with my surrender, I found peace.

James had been driving to College Station from Houston twice a week for over a month. One Sunday afternoon in August, at a little park near the campus, I asked James if he wanted to marry me. I told you. I was a hopeless romantic; also hopelessly impatient. It only took seconds for my question to sink in. Then he gave his answer: an emphatic and enthusiastic, "Yes, of course. I'd be crazy not to. I love you with all my heart. Will you marry me?"

I've never let him forget that I proposed to him. But, Hey. I had places to go and things to do. And I was not entirely confident that marriage was in this "confirmed" bachelor's plans. But it was, and it was in God's plans.

Psalm 18:20 *(The Message)* says, "God made my life complete when I placed all the pieces before Him." On a beautiful Fall day, November 9, 1957, we were married, surrounded by those we loved best: parents, siblings, nieces, nephews, cousins, dear friends, and a host of James' Shell Oil Company colleagues. Two of my closest friends from Nursing School were my bridesmaids; two others provided the music.

It was a beautiful sacred ceremony in our lovely church worship center in Houston, Texas. It was all that I could have dreamed of – and more. That day, when James and I traditionally promised to love one another "for better, for worse, for richer, for poorer, in sickness and in health, till death do us part," we meant every word of that promise. We still do.

Even though James doesn't remember any of this love story I've shared with you, he still says every night at bedtime, "Remember, till death do us part." I, on the other hand, remember every detail. I keep those memories tucked safely away in my heart.

"James, thank you for loving me all these years; for making me feel like a 'Princess'; for reminding me, even now, several times a day, "I love you from the bottom of my heart." That is the one thing that you consistently remember. Along with our faith in God, it is the one constant in our lives—the glue that holds us together on this long journey."

Chapter 3

Dance Lessons from My Mother

Cherish the gift – God's plan.
Cherish the plan – God's promise.
Cherish the promise – God's love.
Cherish the love – God's fulfillment.
~Lucy

The lessons my wise mother taught me had to do with the wonderful "dance" of a happy marriage, the beautiful rhythm of two people in love. She and my father, at least in my hearing, never said a cross, hurtful or critical word to one another. Theirs was a love story to emulate. My father treated my mother like a queen. My parents worked hard at keeping their love and their dreams alive. They were an inspiration to me.

The week before my wedding, my mother who was a poet and an artist, wrote me a letter containing great truths from her marriage. These were her words, her "dance lessons" for me:

♥ Cherish James with all your heart and tell him you love him every day. Realize that he is a gift from God. Keep your home and yourself neat, clean, and attractive so he will always be proud of you. (This is one of the best ways to show your love for him.) When it is possible, be home to greet him when he arrives from work.

♥ Listen to him. When he comes home, ask him about his day and listen with your ears and your heart. Do this before you unload your problems and frustrations of the day. This will be much harder than you think, but the rewards are great.

♥ Admire and respect him. Ephesians 5:33 reads, "Each of you also must love his wife as he loves himself, and the wife must respect her husband." Do this by asking for and valuing his opinions, praising him to others, and trusting his judgment and decisions.

♥ Show your love and appreciation for him. Encourage him. Leave love notes where he will find them. Praise him when he does a good job and refrain from criticizing him when he fails. Never knowingly wound his spirit; build him up at every opportunity. Remember, hurtful words stay in the heart forever.

♥ Be his best friend. Plan date nights. Get a babysitter and plan something he likes to do. Encourage him to do things occasionally with his friends, like ball games or fishing. Surprise him on special occasions with candlelight and his favorite meal. (Send the children over to friends for the night.) Be sure he knows that, after God, he is your first love, your first concern.

♥ Pray for him every day. Remember that this partnership requires three people – You, James, and the Lord. Never leave the Lord out, and your life together will be what He planned for you from the beginning of time.

Chapter 4

Dancing for Joy on Our Road to the Future

Step
by step
by step
Our joyful dance to the future begins
Feeling more joy than my heart can contain,
My "butterfly-dance" through life ends.
From now on I'll dance with my sweetheart,
Building beautiful memories of our love;
Blessed by the love and joy we share:
Gifts from our Father above.
~Lucy

The day after our wedding, on our way to Hot Springs, Arkansas, James and I stopped at a quiet little roadside park. We rejoiced in the beautiful, perfect Fall morning; crisp November air; trees filled with the breathtaking beauty of red and gold leaves; joyful bird songs. Love and joy welled up like a fountain in our hearts.

It was Sunday morning, and because we would normally be in church, we had a special time of worship – just the two of us, our first as husband and wife. It was a sweet sacred time of worship there in that beautiful tabernacle of nature. I read a scripture. We sang our favorite hymn, and James prayed. Almost fifty-two years later, we had another remarkable, sweet worship time – just the two of us and God (I'll share that story later). I don't remember all the details of that first Sunday service together, but I will never forget my joy and the feeling of completeness. That morning my happiness was almost too much to contain. The beauty around us and inside me was tangible. I could taste it; feel it; touch it. I felt that my heart would burst with love for James and gratitude to God the Father for this gift of love.

I'm not making this up. These are not just pretty words. These feelings and memories are as real today as they were that day, November 10, 1957. It was the end of my ceaseless "butterfly dance" through life. It was the beginning of a joyful dance into the future where endless adventures were waiting.

Would our world always be as beautiful as it was that day? Would my heart always almost burst with love for James as it did that day? Would joy always well up until I felt that my heart was not large enough to contain it? Only God knew the answers to these questions that day. Only God knows the future. I do know this – that day we placed all of our future days and years in His strong, loving, powerful hands.

The days that followed that perfect Sunday morning were very near to what I imagined Heaven to be like. They were days filled with the beauty of the Ozark Mountains in the Fall Season. They were filled with joy, contentment, and completeness. Our journey into the future had begun. And I began looking at life, not through rose-colored glasses, but through "Christ-colored" glasses.

Chapter 5

Traveling Light and Carefree

How much more joy can two hearts hold
When they are already overflowing
With love and contentment, hope and peace,
Blessings God is freely bestowing?
With thankful hearts, Lord, we give You glory
With gratitude, we give You praise,
And, together, make this solemn commitment:
To serve You faithfully all of our days.
~Lucy

In spite of a wonderful, joy-filled honeymoon in Arkansas, we were anxious to get home to our new little apartment. There were very few nice apartment complexes in Houston, Texas in 1957. We were fortunate to find a brand new garage apartment down the block from where James lived. I had been living there for almost a month before our wedding. I am ashamed to admit that I was scared to death after James left every evening to go down the street to his apartment.

After James left each night, I would drag everything I could move against the locked door before going to bed. I had never before spent a single night by myself. I learned in those few weeks to trust God as I had never trusted Him before. I became well acquainted with the Psalms, which I read every night at bedtime: "The Lord watches over all who love Him." (Psalm 145:20); "Keep me safe, 0 God, for, in You, I take refuge", (Psalm 16:1); "I sought the Lord, and He answered me; He delivered me from all of my fears." (Psalm 34:4). I was ashamed of my fears; afraid God would think I didn't have faith in His ability to watch over me. (I had the same feeling the day in August of 2009, when, because of James' sundowner's (night fears), I had a security system installed in our home on Rainbow Bend). But God was patient and faithful during those days. It truly was a special time of learning to lean entirely on Him. He knew how much I would need that lesson for all the days and years ahead.

Little did we know when we arrived home, tired and hungry, anxious to get unpacked, that we would first need to unpack our bathroom. It was filled to the ceiling with crumpled newspaper. By the time we had gathered all this paper into ten or twelve large trash bags, we were exhausted and covered from head to foot with black newsprint ink. (As I am writing these words, I am reminded that now, fifty-two years later, I spend a part of every day wiping black fingerprints off my white kitchen counter and black newsprint ink off of James' fingers each time he reads that day's newspaper. He sometimes reads it eight or ten times —or more. He loves reading the newspaper.) As we closed the last bag, the culprits, our "best friends," Win and Lettie, and James' niece, Paula, came up the stairs, carrying food and my apartment key, which my "fun-loving" mother had so generously supplied. By then, I was a real mess, my face streaked with tears and black ink, but soon we were all laughing hysterically. We were paying for all of James' tricks played during his bachelor years on his friends at their weddings. I think we could call things even that day.

Thus began our wonderful, carefree life together. I read recently a beautiful thought: "Happy marriages begin when we marry the ones we love, and they blossom when we love the ones we marry.[4] Our love and our marriage did blossom.

Even though God had chosen a different plan for my life, a plan that did not include a mission field in Africa, I had no trouble finding a place of service with James, wherever we were. We had made a commitment of servanthood to God at the beginning of our marriage. From then on we fulfilled our commitment in whatever ministry He chose for us. James' servant heart was an inspiration to me and to everyone who knew him.

---

4   Tom Mullen, Southern Lady, March/April 2010, p. 70.

Now, fast forward to New Year's Eve 1998. Past the purchase of two much loved houses. Past the birth of three wonderful sons. Past the joys and challenges of parenthood and the difficulty of letting go when the time came. Past the acquisition of two beautiful daughters- in-law. Past the gift of three precious grandsons. Past the timely retirement from our chosen professions. Past memorable vacations. Past the sadness at the death of our parents and other loved ones. Past James' successful coronary artery bypass surgery in 1994. Past all of the normal stresses of living in an imperfect world.

During those years James and I never doubted that God was with us through every situation. We were content and our love for one another grew stronger each day until we finally shared one heart.

Chapter 6

Marching Courageously Through the Year 1999

"Be strong and courageous. Do not be
terrified, do not be discouraged, for
the Lord, your God, will be with
you wherever you go"
(Joshua 1:9).

"One thing I do – it is my aspiration:
forgetting what lies behind and straining
forward to what lies ahead, I press on
toward the goal to win the [supreme and
heavenly] prize to which God in
Christ Jesus is calling us upward.
Only let us hold true to what we
have already attained and walk and order
our lives by that"
(Philippians 3:13, 14, 16 AMP).

My Journal – 1:15 A.M. January 1, 1999

*"Earlier tonight, James and I were upstairs at David and
Pam's house. We were doing what we love best – entertaining
our grandsons. We had a picnic and then played games with
Adam and Matthew, age six, and Micah, age two. They
finally gave up and went to sleep. James and I then watched
New Year's Eve festivities on television.*

*Adam's parents, David and Pam, and Matthew and Micah's
parents, Matt and Roxann were downstairs with Tim and
his girlfriend, Kathy. They were having a "dress-up, grown-*

ups-only" party. It was a wise, safe alternative to going out for the evening. After cleaning up the kitchen, they sat down to watch television. They always enjoy being together, and having Tim and Kathy here from San Antonio for part of the holidays is a real treat. We all love Kathy, who has been dating Tim for over a year. She is teaching in San Antonio and staying with Tim's friends who are members of his church.

At 11:45, I said, "James, it's almost midnight. Let's go downstairs and welcome in the New Year with our children."

He said, "I can't go, I don't want to. You go." No amount of begging or persuading would change his mind. Completely baffled, I went downstairs to tell the others that James wasn't feeling well and that I would stay upstairs with him. Within minutes, the sound of fireworks and horns blowing signaled the beginning of a New Year, the Year 1999.

I gently kissed a somber, subdued James and wished him a Happy New Year. It was almost as if a stranger had taken over my usually strong, happy, loving husband's body and personality. Suddenly, I couldn't help wondering what this New Year would bring into our safe, secure, blessed-beyond-measure lives.

We got home shortly after midnight. James was exhausted and he went straight to bed. I, on the other hand, I'm wide-awake wondering what is going on with James. I start to pray but don't know what to pray. Instead, I say, "Father, please help us." I'll try to sleep now. (Lucy)

James slept in on New Year's Day (a first for him), but I was up early. I'm the designated "roast beef, mashed potatoes, black-eyed peas, cornbread" preparer. Pam's parents came for lunch and brought potato salad and pecan pie, James' favorite.

The men, as usual, watched as many ball games as possible, and the women cooked, cleaned, and kept up with the children. James, the captain of his high school football team and the recipient of an athletic scholarship to SMU, loves football. Today, he seemed more like himself but appeared tired. I could tell that he was enjoying the camaraderie of friends and family. For that, I was so grateful. At the end of the first day of the New Year, I could say that it had been a good day, a blessed day.

After Tim and Kathy left the next day to go to their homes in San Antonio, James just sat in his recliner. Once again, he was moody and seemed depressed. I finally sat down beside him and asked him what he was feeling – why he was so sad. His answer surprised me. "I thought Tim would ask Kathy to marry him during the holidays. I thought he would give her an engagement ring for Christmas."

As I thought about his explanation, I realized that he was afraid; afraid that we might lose Kathy. She was a perfect fit for our family; a perfect match for Tim. I assured James that we had raised smart sons and that Tim knew what he was doing. Which he did. What bothered me was that James' reaction to all this made no sense.

The last week of January 1999, in a most romantic, pre-arranged setting in San Antonio, Tim proposed to Kathy, and she said, "yes." He had been strategically planning this for some time. James and I were both thrilled with this fantastic news. All parents want to know that their children have found the right person to share their life.

The first day of February 1999, I was upstairs putting away the last of the Christmas decorations when I heard the doorbell. I walked out onto the upstairs balcony and saw James talking to a young man in our entry hall.

James said, "Honey, there's someone here to see you." Puzzled, I went downstairs and greeted a very nice young man. He told me his name and handed me his card. He said, "I have an appointment with your husband. I'm a financial advisor, and I'd like to discuss with you and your husband some investment opportunities."

I knew I had not made the appointment, and when I asked James if he had done so, he looked 'blank'. The young man, Paul, looked puzzled and a little uncomfortable, so I invited him to sit down. As he opened his Daily Planner and read the name of the person he had spoken with, I realized that James had indeed made the appointment. I was beginning to sense that this might be a "Divine appointment." In the years that followed, Paul and I always agreed that it must have been God who sent him to our door that day.

For the next eight years, this young man diligently and brilliantly handled our financial affairs. On that first visit, he discussed with James and me our philosophy and goals concerning our savings. He discussed the wisdom of having a Revocable Living Trust rather than a traditional Will. He also advised us to consider Long Term Care Insurance. Within a week, we had started the process to accomplish both suggestions and soon our Revocable Living Trust was established. With his help, we also found the appropriate investment strategy for our savings. I highly recommend that everyone find a financial coach they can trust to handle their financial affairs.

God knew the importance of all this long before it happened. Looking back, even after all this time, I realize that He was, as usual, meeting our needs at exactly the right time. Our Heavenly Father, in His infinite wisdom, knew that someday soon we would need a Medical and Financial Power of Attorney and Living Wills. He knew that the time was coming when James would be unable to understand and process all the paperwork involved.

On February 15, 1999, James, as usual, gathered all the information needed to prepare our income taxes, something he had done routinely and effortlessly for the past forty-one years of our marriage. He sat down that morning with all the forms, looked at them, shuffled them a few times, then looked at me. There was confusion and fear in his eyes. He said, "I don't know how to do this. We'll have to find someone to help us with it this year." There was fear in my heart. I thought, "What is happening to my brilliant, financially astute husband? What is happening to our calm, secure and stable life?"

On the evening of February 21, 1999, a Sunday, James and I were returning from a funeral home where we had attended the viewing for an old friend. James, who always drove, suddenly almost hit the left-side curb then swerved into the right lane, almost hitting a car. He gained control, but again began having trouble staying in his lane. I asked him to pull over so that I could drive home. He explained that the lanes "kept moving" and "would not stay straight."

This was my first real wake-up call that something was seriously wrong with James. The first thing Monday morning, February 22, I called our Internist who told me to bring James in immediately. After taking a brief history and doing a quick exam, he called a Neurologist in the same building. As busy as she was, she agreed to see James that day, a real miracle. We went straight upstairs to her office.

Over the course of the next week, James had an MRI, a CAT Scan and, on March 2, 1999, a sleep-deprived EEG. The EEG would reveal that, sometime in the past, James had suffered a left frontal lobe stroke. This particular part of the brain controls logic and reasoning, which would explain some of James' unusual emotional changes. However, because James had two older sisters who had died after suffering with Alzheimer's for ten years, the Neurologist ordered Psychological testing. After a couple of hours, she concluded that the tests did not point to Alzheimer's. She suggested that we continue to consult with James' Cardiologist and that we should make an appointment to see her again in three or four months. Although the news of a past stroke was unsettling, it helped to explain James' depression and frequent anxiety. We were both so relieved that there was no indication of Alzheimer's disease.

In April of 1999, a beautiful gift brought joy into our lives. Brett, our fourth grandson, was born. There was so much joy that day—joy that dispelled some of the anxiety we were experiencing because of James' continuing health problems.

The month of May 1999 was filled with the preparations for Tim and Kathy's upcoming wedding. There was shopping for a new dress for me, long distance arrangements for James' tuxedo, final preparations for the food and flowers for the Rehearsal Dinner James and I were hosting. I was very busy, and the month passed quickly.

The month of June brought the incredibly beautiful wedding. James and I stayed at Kathy's family home in the Dallas area. I was a little apprehensive, aware that being in an unfamiliar setting might be stressful for James. It was. On the way from the wedding rehearsal to the rehearsal dinner we were hosting, James got lost. Because I was not driving, I had not paid close attention to directions. I should have. We finally arrived at the country club where everyone was worried, wondering where we were—the Host and Hostess.

It turned out to be a wonderful party. I could sense, however, that James was very stressed. Getting lost and having to ask for directions embarrassed him and robbed him of some of the joy of the occasion. As we left the club, he seemed a little unsteady and confused. He stumbled while stepping off a curb and fell, hurting his hands (and his pride).

I had to drive home and help him get ready for bed. We were both frazzled. And we still have a wedding the next day. Thankfully, James slept well. I, on the other hand, tried to process what had happened in the past few hours. It was the first time in almost forty-two years of marriage that I had seen James helpless and not in control. Here we were, away from home, out of our comfort zone. I was suddenly faced with the reality that this could be preview of what our future might be. Again, my prayer was, "Father, please help us."

The wedding was perfect in every way. James, the "perfect" man, looked very handsome in his tux. So did our three sons and our three oldest grandsons.

The next morning, James and I left and made the trip home to Houston safely. We saw his Neurologist on June 29, 1999, at which time she recommended that we sell our two-story house, which held so many wonderful memories. She felt this was advisable because of James' stroke. She also shared that, at the end of June, she was no longer on our Insurance plan. With the help of our primary care physician, we made an appointment for July with a new Neurologist.

On July 22, 1999, my sixty-fifth birthday, we saw James' new doctor. He had received James' medical history from the previous doctor, and we went over it with him. After a brief assessment, this Neurologist decided to give James another Mental State Examination, as he referred to it. While he administered the test, I tried to relax, to not be afraid. I thought of all the times in the Bible when God said to His people, "Do not fear. Do not be afraid. Do not be anxious. When you pass through the waters, I will be with you. Do not be terrified. Do not be discouraged. Wait for the Lord, be strong." All these verses, these promises, these commands played in my mind like a recording. They were a tremendous comfort, and I realized that God's Spirit was speaking to me through these familiar verses, pouring hope and courage into my heart and mind.

When the test was completed, the doctor sat quietly for a moment, then he looked at us and said, "I'm so sorry, but given his history and the results of today's test, in my opinion, it's Alzheimer's." Our worst fears had been confirmed. The doctor started him on Aricept that day. "Part Two" tells the story of our thirteen-year journey with Alzheimer's disease.

Through the next few months, to the casual observer, James appeared perfectly normal. He was taking Aricept without any side effects. I knew, however, that he was having increasing difficulty making decisions. Also, there was a gradual but persistent loss of logic and reasoning.

In August of 1999, at the suggestion of James' doctor, we prepared to sell our two-story home on an oversized lot. We found a Realtor, had a enormous garage sale, and staged our house for showing.

In September and October, we were consumed with finding exactly the right new home for us. I tell the story of our "miracle house," in "Part Two." We found it the first of October.

November 5, 1999, we moved into our new home. I was exhausted, but so relieved to be finally settled. The responsibility of making most of the decisions had taken me out of my comfort zone. Thanksgiving in our beautiful new home was wonderful. All the boys and their wives, children, and in-laws joined us for a memorable, joyous time of thanksgiving for God's incredible blessings.

December, 1999, as usual, was a whirlwind of activity. Christmas was filled with joy, celebration, and unusual peace in the midst of the gathering darkness of dementia. As we ended the year 1999, I couldn't help remembering how the year had begun. I prayed for God's guidance and presence in the year ahead. Knowing that God is always faithful gave me hope for the year to come.

Should Your Memories Fade

Should your memories fade, but mine remain
To remember our story of all that's gone before,
I'll be the guardian of these memories so priceless,
Precious mind-pictures to cherish forevermore.

Should your memories fade, but mine remain
To remember a courtship so special and rare,
I'll tell how we miraculously met and found love,
A love story I'm always ready to share.

Should your memories fade, but mine remain
To remember our wedding vows, commitments spoken,
I'll store carefully my memories of that November day
When we made those vows to keep, never to be broken.

Should your memories fade, but mine remain
To remember breathless joy at our journey's start,
I'll write of how step-by-step we began this journey
That has brought us so close, we now share one heart.

Should your memories fade, but mine remain
To remember how wonderful my hand felt in yours,
I'll relate how blessed and cherished I felt
To be sharing with you love that still endures.

Should your memories fade, but mine remain
To remember the wonder of babies and growing boys,
I'll recall laughter and loss that are part of our history,
A bitter-sweet mingling of sorrows and joys.

Should your memories fade, but mine remain
To remember our love, unchanged through the years,
I'll guard well our life's tapestry woven with love
That I will see clearly while smiling through my tears.

~Lucy

PART TWO

Our Journey into the Unknown of Alzheimer's Disease—A Guided Tour

The Lord has been my Shepherd
and Guide all my Life.
Psalm 23

A Guided Tour

Today, I'm lost in this wilderness,
This valley of confusion and sorrow,
Unable to see the path once so clear
Or the promise of hope for tomorrow.
So I'll rest here awhile, down on my knees.
While I wait for my Guide, I'm praying.
Then I realize he's been here all the time,
And I hear His dear voice saying,
"You don't have to see tomorrow's path;
Just this day, this moment, this minute.
Follow Me, my child, I am the way.
By faith now walk you in it."

~Lucy

Chapter 7

Our Journey Begins

Some moments in life, some words, we never forget.
Like fossils imprisoned in ancient rocks, they are
embedded in our memory forever.

On July 22, 1999, my sixty-fifth birthday, at 12:30 P.M., I heard these words from the mouth of James' neurologist: "It's Alzheimer's." They were the words I had begged God we would never hear. These dreaded words were like an arrow that pierced my heart. In an instant, they forever changed the way we would view our future. Our safe, carefree, predictable, productive life would never again be the same. At first, I couldn't say anything. I just sat there.

James turned to me, his blue eyes clear and untroubled. He took my hand and said, "It's going to be okay." I wasn't sure that he processed all that had been said that day. I knew that he was exhausted from all the questions and activities of the testing. Although I was devastated, I managed to "keep it together" for his sake.

The doctor talked to us for a little while, then gave us some samples of the wonderful drug, Aricept. After discussing with us the possible side effects, he walked us out to the front desk where we made another appointment. As we left the office and went out into the warmth of that July day, I felt fragile and cold. I wondered if I would ever feel safe and warm again. Even though the sun was shining, I felt as if we were walking into a dark tunnel with no light at the end. Our journey with Alzheimer's disease had begun.

Because James was tired, I decided to drive. I asked if he wanted to stop to eat, but he kept saying, "Let's go home. Can we just go home?" Once we arrived, I fed James a late lunch, then watched as he settled into his recliner in the den for a nap. He was asleep within seconds.

I could hardly wait to get to my "Bethel", a blue chair in the living room, my retreat from the world, my "Sanctuary" where I spend time with God every day. There on my knees, I gave into my despair. This was not the way I had planned to celebrate my birthday.

As I knelt there, I didn't try to reason away my grief. Actually, I felt that it was appropriate. With two words: "It's Alzheimer's", our world had fallen apart. Although there had been some troubling "indicators" in the previous months, I had pushed them aside attributing them to the left frontal lobe stroke James had suffered sometime in the recent past. Now there was no rationalizing, no denying the truth. Because of James' two sisters, I was well acquainted with Alzheimer's.

I knew that, for now, there was no cure for this disease – no hope that James would get better or go into "remission." I was faced with the stark truth that the rest of James' life would be lived with a "terminal illness." It is an illness that would gradually rob us of everything that was dear and familiar: our shared memories, our relationship and companionship, the very essence of James Dishongh—my brilliant, godly husband, my lover, my best friend.

Facing that "terminal" diagnosis that day was the hardest thing I ever did. I knew that our only hope was our faith and trust in God, our Heavenly Father. That afternoon, with a broken heart, I turned to Him for comfort. I needed this private time with my Father in this special place. I knew that He is the "Mender-of-broken hearts", and I laid my broken heart at His feet. Somehow I sensed that this was the first of many days in the months and years ahead that I would spend on my knees pouring out my heart to Him. I had no way of knowing that it would be thirteen years. I got up feeling encouraged and comforted. After this quiet time of meditation with God the Father, I realized that, even though the "walls" of my safe, secure life had come crashing down that day, the "foundation", my faith, was still strong and intact.

After a light supper of cereal and fruit, James and I sat down together on the couch in the den. I didn't turn on the TV. I was exhausted, physically and emotionally. James reached for the remote, then hesitated. He looked at me, then put his arms around me, holding me close. It was just what I needed. Holding back tears and gathering my courage, I said, "Honey, did you understand what the doctor told us today?" I held my breath as I waited for his answer.

James kissed me on the forehead and said, "You're not having a very happy birthday. I'm sorry." I explained to him that we would celebrate my birthday with the children on the weekend.

My question hung in the air, waiting for an answer. It was like an elephant in the room. It couldn't be ignored. I realize now that we both dreaded opening that "door", facing the reality of what we knew was waiting on the other side. After what seemed like an eternity, James looked into my eyes and said, "I understood everything the doctor said. I guess I already knew what he would say. I know that I don't always feel like myself. Sometimes I'm confused, and I can't remember where I'm going. I didn't want to admit to you that I was having problems because I knew you'd worry" (Of course, I was already worried.).

I don't know whether I was more shocked or more relieved by his answer. Probably a lot of both. I hugged James so tight, and we cried together. It was such a relief to share this heavy burden – to know that we could comfort one another. I know that isn't always the case. But then, not everyone has a "James" in their life. That night we prayed together and made a commitment to trust God with our future, whatever it held. We went to bed, comforted by one another's strength and our faith in God. We had never once said the word "Alzheimer's."

In the days following James' diagnosis, at times I felt a little like Nick, a character in one of my favorite short stories, "The Battler", by Earnest Hemingway. Nick had been thrown from a boxcar of a moving train. This trauma had left him wounded – scraped and bruised – and, worst of all, stranded and alone in the middle of nowhere.

Eleven years later, an article, *Keeping Faith on the Way to Somewhere*, was printed in *In Touch*[5], January 2011. Jeff Manion writes about Nick's situation, and I quote: "This is the image that comes to mind when I think of people I know who have received disruptive news that has radically reshaped their lives, leaving them dazed and stranded. We always tend to remember where we were when the news came." He goes on to say, "With a single sentence, we're thrown out of normality

---

5   Jeff Manion, *Keeping Faith on the Way to Somewhere*," In Touch, January 2011, p. 29.

and suddenly find ourselves going nowhere in a dark new world." I could have written his every word from personal experience.

I wish I could tell you that living with Alzheimer's got easier, but that would not be true. In this "new world", each day brought with it fear of the unknown. I became almost paranoid. Daily, I found myself watching James for any sign of change. It seemed that I was always waiting for "the other shoe to drop."

In 2009 I read a statement by Max Lucado, "feed your fears and your faith will starve. Feed your faith, and your fears will." After reading that and thinking about the truth of it, I recalled asking God in 1999 to replace my fear with a stronger faith. As the days turned into weeks and the weeks into years, my fears were gradually replaced with a growing faith, one I was desperately cultivating and fertilizing with increased prayer and Bible study.

My quiet times with the Lord developed into a deeper intimacy with Him. He became my refuge and strength. Through His Word, he encouraged me to be strong and courageous (*Joshua* 1). He promised to be my Strong Tower to which I could run anytime I needed help. I began to talk to Him, day and night.

As time went by, James and I began to adjust our thinking to accommodate this, our "new normal." We began to find a "rhythm" for living with Alzheimer's. This disease had disrupted our safe, predictable life, radically changing it in many ways. With one dreaded word, "Alzheimer's," we had embarked on a journey where everything would eventually change – our plans, our dreams, our ministry, our vocabulary and even our home.

We soon discovered, in the midst of our heartache, that there is "one light shining in a dark time as you wait for daybreak and the rising of the Morning Star in your hearts" (2 Peter 1:19 *The Message*). That "light" refers to God's voice. We realized that this life with Alzheimer's, this journey that we had begun, would need to be traveled with a deep awareness of God's Presence.

James and I knew that we would need God's guidance every step of the way. Therefore, with as much faith as we could "muster", we surrendered our future to God and asked Him to be our Guide into this frightening unknown world of Alzheimer's disease. As always, He answered our prayer.

As weeks turned into months and months into years, instead of asking the Lord, "Why?" I began asking Him, "What do you want me to do with the lessons You are teaching me through this tragedy of Alzheimer's?"

Though I did not audibly hear His voice, through His Spirit within me, the Lord said, "Write them down. There are others who have started, or will be starting, their journey with Alzheimer's. They will need to know what you are learning as you walk with Me. I will send my Spirit to guide and direct you as you tell Our story – yours and Mine."

I found the journal I had begun writing in March of 1999 during the long days of testing that would reveal the left frontal lobe stroke James had suffered. As I experienced each "breakdown" and each "break-through," I began documenting my feelings as honestly and transparently as possible.

There is a scripture, Psalm 119:28, which is underlined and highlighted in my Bible: "My soul is weary with sorrow; strengthen me according to your Word."

Every time God revealed Himself to me through His Word, I wrote how His promises gave me the courage and strength I needed for that day. In that same *Psalm* 119 are these words, in verses *forty-nine* and *fifty*. "Remember your word to your servant, for you have given me hope. My comfort in my suffering is this: Your promise preserves my life." How awesome that my gracious Father would reveal to me these inspired words spoken by the Psalmist to our Father.

During those days, God's promises did "preserve my life." I didn't want to waste any of the pain and grief I was feeling. Neither did I want to waste the wonderful knowledge that God was walking with me and blessing me each step I took. I didn't want to forget anything He was teaching me along the way.

On our forty-second anniversary, November 9, 1999, James, and I went to dinner to celebrate. As we talked, I began reminiscing about how we met through a "blind date and about the tornado that hit Kyle Field at College Station on our second date. I suddenly realized that James remembered very little of this special time in our life together. Until now, I had not been concerned about James' long-term memory— only his now obvious short-term memory loss. (After dinner, James couldn't remember where we had parked the car at the restaurant).

The next morning, I sat down with my journal. I began to go back into my memories of our life together from that first "mirror encounter" to the present. As I began to write, I prayed that I would never forget a single detail.

I knew in my heart that James was already forgetting. That's why I began writing all of our story. I wanted to be able to share with him my written, preserved memories. I felt that writing them down would give me strength for what lay ahead in what would become our "new normal." Also, I wanted our children and anyone else (especially you, Beloved Caregiver) who might read them, to be encouraged by my documentation of God's faithfulness in our lives – then and now. The result is the book you now hold in your hand.

The Journey Begins

Struggling to breathe,
Surrounded by night,
I'm awake in the darkness,
Longing for light.
Then I hear my Father say,
"My child, do not fear.
I love you so much,
I will always be here."
Calmed by his presence,
My heart breathes a prayer.
I awake in the morning
And find Him waiting there.
~Lucy

(Written the week after we moved into our "miracle house" on Rainbow Bend Drive.)

Chapter 8

Risking the Journey into the Unknown

Life is full of risks. Every time we drive onto a busy freeway, we're taking a risk. Every time businessmen and women board a plane to fly to a required conference or meeting, they're taking a risk. They have no choice. They must trust the skill of the pilot and the safety of the plane to get them to their destination. The same is true of many situations in life over which we have no control.

"Stop this gurney. I want to get off. I've changed my mind." As a surgical nurse, I sometimes heard words to this effect from my patients.

I know the feeling. More than once in the early years of our journey with Alzheimer's, I mentally said, "Stop this journey. I want to get off. I've changed my mind. I'm afraid."

Just as I reassured my patients that they could trust the skill of their surgeon, God reassured me that I could trust Him with my fears and anxiety. He reminded me that when I was walking in difficult places, He would give me the strength and courage to face whatever I would encounter on the path – not all at once, but day by day, step by step.

James' favorite Scripture passage was, "Trust in the Lord with all your heart and lean not on your own understanding; in all your ways acknowledge him and he will make your paths straight." Those verses, Proverbs 3:5-6, became my life verses, also. They are written across my heart and engraved on my mind.

Even so, when the Lord asked James and me to follow Him into the unknown, uncharted territory of Alzheimer's disease, I was terrified. I knew in my heart that God never asks us to do anything for which He has not already equipped us. I also knew that He never allows anything to happen to His children that has not first been filtered through His love and grace. And, if it does come, He always has a purpose for it.

I knew all of this. It wasn't God that I doubted. It was my own strength and courage that I questioned. I had been, until now, sheltered from much of the "ugliness and hardships" of life, and my faith was essentially untested. I wanted so much to face this time of testing with a strong faith. I'm not saying that I believe that God intentionally places tragedy in our lives to test our faith. I do believe, along with the apostle Paul, "We are assured and know that all things work together and are (fitting into a plan) for good to and for those who love God and are called according to (His) design and purpose" (Romans 8:28 AMP).

Much of my fear came from the fact that I had seen what Alzheimer's had done to the mind, body, and life of each of James' two older sisters. I had witnessed the heartache and grief of their families. For this reason, the one thing for which I consistently prayed was that God would spare James and me from this terrible disease. I couldn't understand why God had chosen this path for us. Why had He chosen not to spare us from the very thing I feared the most? I struggled with this for days.

On the face of things, James' illness made little sense to me. He was a devout servant of the Lord whom he loved with all his heart. He was a man of great strength, courage, and integrity. He was bright, loving, and funny. He was an excellent husband, father, and grandfather. After forty years of faithful, loyal service to Shell Oil Company, he was enjoying every minute of his well-earned retirement.

One day I knelt and poured out my struggles and questions to God. I prayed, "Father, I've tried never to question Your divine plans, but 'Why James?' I'm trying so hard to understand." In my spirit, I heard God's answer: "Why not James, Lucy? Because of the years you and James have served Me and walked with Me, you two can be a tremendous witness for Me to a watching world. I have allowed you to walk this path for such a time as this – to be a light for Me in the dark world of dementia and to be a testimony to My faithfulness. I will be walking every step with you. Trust Me with all your heart and don't try to understand it all now."

I realized that God was speaking to me through the words of James' life verse. As I knelt at my "Bethel", letting God pour out His message to me, my troubled heart knelt, too. I surrendered my fears and all my future days to my Father, making a commitment to honor Him with this tragedy and to trust Him with our future.

I wish I could tell you that there is an easy way to face a future with an illness that holds no hope of a cure or even remission during your loved one's lifetime. But that wouldn't be true. There were times when the reality of what we were facing caused such pain I thought I wouldn't survive. There were times when I hurt too much to cry.

As time passed, however, I realized that even gut-wrenching grief does not take God by surprise. His Word never lies to us by telling us that our lives will be easy. It does, however, promise us that God will never leave us or forsake us.

The Apostle Paul was a perfect example of one who daily lived out his faith despite difficult circumstances and dangers. He often referred to his life as a "race." I thought of him often in the early days following James' diagnosis. Like him, my desire was to run my race with my eyes on Jesus. I knew this would inspire me and keep me looking forward. Therefore, anytime I wanted to give up, I ran to Jesus. He invited me to run with Him, to follow Him, to draw strength from Him, and to rest in Him. I heard His invitation through God's Word: "Come to me, all you who are weary and burdened, and I will give you rest." (Matthew 11:28); "Come, follow me" (Matthew 4:19).

With Jesus running with me, I found the stamina and the courage to keep running. He knew that without His presence and encouragement, I might not be able to face the risks one encounters on an unfamiliar path. I was so grateful for the realization that He knows all about Alzheimer's disease and that He already knew what we would experience during our journey.

As I'm writing, I'm thinking about how wonderful it is to have this inner peace and strength that I have experienced daily throughout our journey. I realize that Jesus has been my guide and "running partner" since that day in January of 1954, when I invited Him into my heart. Without His constant presence in my life since that day, I would not be who I am today. I certainly would not have been equipped to walk this journey – to run this "race." I'm very sure I would not have finished well.

In my spirit, I can still hear Jesus saying, "Lucy, don't run ahead of Me. You may lose your way and miss things I want to teach you. Don't lag too far behind, trying to hold onto the past. Just run with Me and like Me, you will be victorious."

I do believe that God entrusted me with the responsibility to demonstrate His grace to those watching from the sidelines as James and I began this journey in July of 1999. Through our response to this tragedy, I wanted to demonstrate that God's grace is sufficient for our needs; that our whole faith-life was risking everything on God's grace.

This was the message I wanted to send to a watching world:

I want my life, no matter what the circumstances, to count for God's Kingdom.

I want my example to encourage others.

I want my faith to inspire those watching.

I want my suffering, my pain, to identify me with Christ.

I want my every action to bring honor and glory to God.

Max Lucado, in *Grace for the Moment*, reminds us, "You can't lose your balance if you never climb. You can take the safe route. Or, you can hear the voice of adventure, follow God's impulses. Make a difference."[6]

At the beginning of this 'Journey", I certainly didn't think of it as "an adventure." I did, however, want to follow God's "impulses", His "calling", and make a difference.

---

6   Max Lucado, Grace tor the Moment, J. Countryman, Division of Thomas Nelson, Inc., Nashville, Tennessee; p. 314.

James and I decided that we wanted to be like Abraham and Sarah. Together, we read God's call to them in Genesis 12:1-2, "The Lord had said to Abram, "Leave your country, your people and your father's household and go to the land I will show you. I will make you into a great nation, and I will bless you; I will make your name great, and you will be a blessing."

Even though our "calling" was different, we wanted to be obedient, just as they were. They acted in faith. They took a risk, not knowing where they were going. They trusted God for the journey and the destination.

The times that James and I spent together in those early years, praying and reading God's Word, are priceless memories for me. James was so precious, and his faith was so strong, even though Alzheimer's was, step by step, day by day, robbing him of logic and reasoning. We agreed that we wanted to continue to be a blessing to our family, our friends and all that we would meet along the way.

Looking back at our life before Alzheimer's and to the present, I realize that the same God who walked with Abraham and Sarah was walking with us then and continued to walk with us throughout our thirteen-year journey. God is still walking with me now.

I am fully convinced that God honored our risk-taking faith. He had known every detail of the future before it happened. Our limited knowledge continually drove us to depend entirely on God's leadership. Because the path into the "unknown" of Alzheimer's was unfamiliar to us, God faithfully guided us.

Psalm 1 in *The Message,* tells us: "The Lord watches over the way of the righteous. God charts the road you take."

The greatest comfort for James and me, as we began this journey into "alien country," was the assurance that we would never be walking alone; that God would always be with us to guide us and to protect us.

Risking the Journey

We're risking this journey into uncharted land,
By faith, we're surrendering to God's plan.

We'll seek His face each step, each mile,
And be encouraged by His loving smile.

Instead of trusting our strength, our pride,
We'll ask God for His back on which to ride.

We'll let Him carry us and set the pace,
While we rest in His awesome, amazing grace.

~Lucy and James

James helped me write this, February 1, 2000.
He selected the scripture below.

"Do not be anxious about anything
but in everything, by prayer and petition,
with thanksgiving, present
your request to God,
and the peace of God which transcends
all understanding will guard your hearts
and minds in Christ Jesus"
(Philippians 4:6-7).

Faith never knows where it is
being led, but it knows and loves
the one who is leading.
~Oswald Chambers

Chapter 9

Introducing the Tour Guides

In October of 2002, James and I took a chartered bus trip, a guided tour of the East Coast to see the fall foliage. It was a trip James and I always had planned to take, but we ran out of time. I knew this would probably be our last opportunity for a real vacation together. We traveled with dear friends from our previous church. These longtime friends promised to help me with James. The men volunteered to help with our luggage and to take James to the men's room during rest stops.

This was my first guided tour, and I loved it. After three years of taking care of the house, the car, the bills, and many of James' needs, I needed someone else to make decisions, plans, and arrangements – even if just for fifteen days. I desperately needed nurturing and pampering. I loved having someone tell me what to do, where and when to eat, where to sleep. For fifteen long, wonderful days, I let someone else do the driving, make all the decisions, be in control. I appreciated it. I welcomed it.

As I'm writing, I'm thinking about how this parallels our journey with Alzheimer's, our "guided tour," with God as our excellent Tour Guide and with loving friends to help along the way. I learned on that trip that the Tour Guide is of primary importance to the safety, comfort, success, and enjoyment of any trip.

This is a perfect time to introduce the Tour Guides for our journey with Alzheimer's. Our Tour Guides are part of the Godhead, which consists of three distinct persons:

✝ God the Father

✝ God the Son

✝ God the Holy Spirit

Dr. Charles Stanley explains it this way: "All three persons have different roles in our lives, but these roles interrelate: The Father creates a plan; Jesus, the Son, implements the plan; the Holy Spirit administers the plan.[7]

Whether we fully understand this or not, which I don't, it is of utmost importance that we understand that there is only one God. His primary plan for us is salvation, transformation and lives that glorify Him. It is imperative that we get God right.

As travelers, when we are on a tour, it is essential that we continually look at our guide for instructions, directions and help. When we let the guide do his job, we can relax and enjoy the trip.

The same is true of God, and as His Holy Spirit leads us, we can follow Him with complete trust and confidence that He knows the way and the itinerary. By faith in our Guide, we can live one day at a time and walk through doors as He opens them for us. With God's guidance, we can confidently walk in His best and rest in His grace every day, every step of our journey.

The Triune God, our Tour Guide, has all the attributes and credentials we could ask for – and more.

> ✝ He is a "person" (Exodus 20:1-6). We are made in his image. He has feelings, such as anger, love, and jealousy.

> ✝ He is "Spirit" (John 4:22-24). He has no limitations. He can be everywhere at all times. His Spirit lives within us as believers. Therefore, we can experience His presence and guidance at any time.

> ✝ He is "eternal"(Psalm 56:19). He has no beginning and no end. He has always been, is now, and always will be.

> ✝ He is "unchangeable" (Hebrew 13:8). He is always constant – the same yesterday, today, and forever.

---

7   Charles Stanley, *In Touch* Magazine, "The Truth About The Trinity", February 2010, 40.

At our moment of salvation, we are provided the perfect Guides for our Christian journey. As we travel this journey, we will need all three: God the Father, God the Son, and God the Holy Spirit.

Think of it. We have a Perfect Father, a Personal Savior, and a Powerful Friend and Comforter.

God's Word clearly and faithfully tells us the attributes of each of our Guides. God Himself tells us His names. As we look at these names, we will realize (and be so grateful for) the personal significance of each one as we walk this difficult journey with Him as our Guide.

Names of God

Elohim - "Creator" (Hebrew, plural) - Genesis 1:1

Yahweh (Jehovah) - "Self-Existent One" - Exodus 3:13-15

Adonai - "Master" - (Hebrew) - "Sovereign Lord

Genesis 15:2

El Shaddai - "All-Sufficient One" - Genesis 17:1-3

El Elyon - "Most High God" ("Leader") - Genesis 14:17-24

Jehovah-Jireh - "Provider" - Genesis 22:14

Jehovah-Shalom - "Giver of Peace" - Judges 6:24

Jehovah-Rophe - "Healer" - Exodus 15:26

Jehovah-Nissi - "Battle Fighter" - Exodus 17:15

Jehovah-Rohi - "Good Shepherd" - Psalm 23:1

Jehovah-Mekadesh - "God Who Sanctifies" - Leviticus 20:8

Jehovah-Sabaoth - "Lord of Hosts" - Psalm 46:7

El Gibbor - "Mighty God" - Isaiah 9:6

Jehovah-Tsidkenu - "The Lord Our Righteousness" -
Jeremiah 23:5-6

El Roi - "God Who Sees" - Genesis 16:1-14

Jehovah - Shammah - "Ever-Present One" - Ezekiel 48:35

Abba - "Father" (Aramic), "Daddy" - Romans 8:15

Jesus - "God Saves" - Matthew 1:21

A SONG FOR JESUS

Jesus, because You are the same
Yesterday, today, and forever,
I can sing in a world that doesn't make sense,
A world that without You, can never
Offer hope for the hurting, the helpless, the weak;
A world that without You is lost,
Needing a Savior, needing a Friend,
One who is willing, no matter the cost,
To give His own life for our freedom from sin,
And who, because of great love
Was born one night into our lost world,
Sent to earth by our Father above.
So I'll be one of the notes that make up the song
That tells of this wondrous love,
A love that endures forever and ever,
And promises to right every wrong.
I'll sing of our Savior, who'll never leave.
He's our Helper who will always be here;
Who says, "I will never forsake you";
Whose assurance removes all my fear.
So, I'll sing my song with gusto,
With confidence and fervor
Because Jesus, You are the same —
Yesterday, today, and forever.

~Lucy

God the Son, Jesus, Emmanuel: God with Us

The day I met Jesus in January of 1954 was the most important day of my life – then, now, and forever.

Since that cold day in 1954, I've never doubted that Jesus is real and that I can trust Him with my life. As the very things that made James so special – his strength, his wisdom, his dependability –were slowly but steadily fading away day by day, I needed something to cling to. More than ever before, I needed something unshakable, dependable, and unchangeable on which to rest. I found that in Jesus.

Life changes; families change; circumstances change; seasons come and go. Only Jesus stays the same. Hebrews 13:8 AMP assures us: "Jesus Christ, the Messiah, (is always) the same, yesterday, today, (yes,) and forever – to the ages."

People leave. Everyone we know will eventually leave us for one reason or another. Only Jesus, the Lord, will never leave us. Hebrews 13:5 promises: "Never will I leave you; never will I forsake you."

God the Father wants to meet our every need – physical, emotional, and spiritual. His goal since the creation of the world has been to reveal what He has done, is doing and will do for us, His creation. Jesus is that revelation. It is crucial, no matter what my circumstances, that I keep a firm grip on what God has revealed to me by the Holy Spirit:

- ✝ Jesus is the centerpiece of all that I believe.
- ✝ Jesus is the cornerstone and foundation of my faith.
- ✝ Jesus is my great High Priest with ready access, at all times, to God the Father.

The book of *Hebrews* teaches me that Jesus is a Priest who is not out of touch with the reality of my life, but is always accessible. He invites me to walk right up to Him and receive His peace, His mercy, and His grace. With Him, I can approach the very throne of God the Father. That's where Jesus is right now, as I'm writing these words.

Romans 8:34 informs us: "Christ Jesus, who died — more than that, who was raised to life — is at the right hand of God and is also interceding for us." The Amplified says that He is " pleading as He intercedes for us."

That truth, that reality is so incredible. At this particular time in my life, I need that kind of love. Jesus' love for me is my haven for hope; my light in the gathering darkness of Alzheimer's. It is my lifeline when I feel that I am drowning in a "river" of tears and sorrow.

"Jesus, thank You for being not only my Savior, but a Friend who "sticks closer than a brother" — and a faithful Guide on this frightening journey.

I will fix my eyes on You. You are not only my Guide, but my destination—The Author and Finisher of my faith. Thank You for running my "race" with me and for inviting me to borrow strength from You anytime I need it."

God the Holy Spirit

God has given a Gift to those of us who have put our faith and trust in Jesus. This precious gift that makes us different from the world is the indwelling presence of the Holy Spirit in our hearts.

Jesus was intimately acquainted with His disciples and knew they would not be able to live a life of faith in their strength. That is why He told them to wait until He had sent them the gift of the Holy Spirit. The promised Holy Spirit came into the world after Jesus ascended to heaven. His purpose was to enable and equip His followers to serve God more effectively.

The same is true of us today. We are powerless without the presence and guidance of the Holy Spirit in our lives. As James and I began our journey into the frightening, unknown future of Alzheimer's disease, we realized we could not walk in our strength and wisdom. From the beginning, we gratefully claimed God's gift to us — the presence of the Holy Spirit.

During these thirteen years, I've learned the secret of living victoriously: Become best friends with the Holy Spirit. He has all the qualities of a best friend:

He is someone I can always lean on.

He helps me make wise decisions.

He is someone with whom I can share my deepest feelings.

He is never too busy to listen.

He always has my best interest at heart.

As caring for James became my main purpose, I often felt cut off from friends and my regular support group, my church. But I was never alone. The Holy Spirit was always with me – loving me, protecting me, guiding me, helping me find the words when I didn't know what to pray. As I opened my Bible each morning, He pointed out scriptures that seemed to be tailor-made for my needs that day.

When my heart was broken, He comforted me. He stayed awake with me through many long nights. He taught me how to rejoice in suffering, how to resist temptation, and how to love in a way the world doesn't understand.

As James and I walked the path God had chosen for us, the Holy Spirit equipped us to thrive and to bear spiritual fruit in our lives, even in the face of the progressive dementia of Alzheimer's.

The reality that the Holy Spirit within a believer never gets dementia was reinforced over and over again by James Dishongh. The love of God flowed through him to everyone he met, even when he didn't know who or where he was. It was amazing to watch this in action.

In the book of *Galatians,* chapter five, Paul lists these virtues, the fruit of the Holy Spirit: love, joy, peace, patience, kindness, goodness, faithfulness, gentleness, and self-control. James was a recipient of these gifts. His life consistently demonstrated these character qualities. His child-like faith and devotion to God, still strong even in his dementia, were a challenge to me and to many others to allow God's Spirit to work in our hearts and lives.

Giver of Gifts: Empowering Spirit

Holy Spirit, when my way is rough and steep,
Keep me from stumbling.
When the path ahead grows dim
And fear distracts me,
Help me to listen to Your guiding voice
Saying, "Walk this way, make Me your choice.
I'll be your Light, your strength, your Guide
Follow Me, walk with Me —Abide."

~Lucy

ℰℐ

"Those who are led by the Spirit of God are Sons of God"
(Romans 8:14).

Chapter 10

A Call to Surrender

Letting Go

There are loved ones we can't live without
But somehow we must let go
To a new world where their memories are fading,
And their steps are growing slow.

To a world where, who they once were,
Is almost forgotten and gone,
But to us who are being left behind,
Our memories of their past live on.

Along with them, we'll begin life anew,
Our steps slowing to match their pace;
Helping them to celebrate daily
Moments of success in their new place.
~Lucy

I wrote these verses October 1, 2011, the day I placed James full-time in Clare Bridge, Brookdale's highly acclaimed Alzheimer's and Dementia Care facility at the Hampton in Pearland.

You may not realize that God's call to surrender to His will – every day—is extremely critical to the success of our journey with Alzheimer's. He wants us to realize that He is all that we need; that we are complete in Him.

God's desire is for us to advance through our adversities rather than getting "stuck" in life's difficult spots because of our pride or self-sufficiency. It is important that we recognize that how we respond to hardship reveals our real character. When we acknowledge that God is sovereign all the time, in good times and bad, we will face difficulties differently. We will be able to face and conquer adversity as we move through it and surrender to God's sovereign will.

This doesn't mean that we will like our situation. It does mean that we will submit to God's desire to mature our faith and make us more like Jesus as a result of our situation. In this spirit of surrender, we will find peace and contentment, even as we face hard times. That's what the apostle Paul was saying to the Christians in Rome in that beautiful passage, Romans 8:28, "And we know that in all things God works for the good of those who love him, who have been called according to his purpose."

Notice the words, "all things." That means that whatever we're facing, even the dreaded dementia of Alzheimer's, God is at work bringing meaning to our tragedy and purpose to our pain. When we look back, I am sure we will realize that we've never before sensed God's love and presence as we did when we came to this "disruptive" moment in our lives.

So many times at the beginning of our journey, I felt bewildered and lost. I would turn in my Bible to my favorite verse: "Be still and know that I am God" (Psalm 46:10). As I read the familiar words, God would remind me that He is the Sovereign Lord of the universe, the One I can trust to be in control of my life, every step of the way.

The practical side of me wanted to take things into my own hands. In my heart, however, I knew that God was telling me to wait and to surrender to His plan for James and me. Deep down, I knew that God's desire was for me to surrender everything in my life to His authority; to let Him "do the driving." He knew that when I did, our journey would be safe and peaceful, even though the road we traveled was rough and dangerous.

You would think that this would be a simple, logical thing to do. I'm very familiar with my "hero" Paul's conversation with God about his "thorn in the flesh." The Bible calls us to a place of surrender, "My grace is enough, it's all you need. My strength comes into its own in your weakness" (2 Corinthians 12:9 *The Message*).

This was God's answer to Paul when he prayed and begged three times for God to remove a frustrating, limiting handicap in his life. In response, Paul made the decision to quit focusing on his problem. He surrendered and let Christ take over, realizing that the weaker he became, the stronger he became. When he "let go", Christ's strength replaced his weakness. Wow. That must have been a tremendous relief to Paul. He said, "I just let Christ take over. And so the weaker I got, the stronger I became" (2 Corinthians 12:10 *The Message*).

Recently I read a devotional from the book, *Jesus Calling*. The author, *Sarah Young*, wrote: "Bring me your weakness and receive My peace. Accept yourself and your circumstances just as they are, remembering that I am sovereign over everything. Do not wear yourself out with analyzing and planning. Instead, let thankfulness and trust be your guides through this day."[8]

We all know that God has not promised freedom from trials and troubles. In her poetry, Annie Johnson Flint reminds us that God has not promised us lives that are easy and carefree. But God has promised that He will give us strength, rest, light, grace, sympathy, and love for each day. This extraordinary woman, orphaned after the deaths of her natural and adoptive parents, had a difficult life. As a young woman, she developed severe, crippling arthritis. From her tragedies, however, came the amazing poetry for which she is known.

Even though I acknowledged and believed all these wonderful truths, I still struggled to "let go." For years I've had a tendency to think that it's my responsibility to make everything "perfect," to believe that I can fix just about anything when I roll up my sleeves and "set my mind" to it. I've always been a natural caregiver. I want to take care of everyone, to right every wrong, to protect my loved ones from worry or hardship.

---

8   Sarah Young, *Jesus Calling* Thomas Nelson, Copyright 2004.

It was not until James' Alzheimer's became a part of my life that I came to recognize my limitations and weakness. As I encountered more and more mountains, I discovered that I could not climb them without God's help, even though I tried very hard. God never gave up on me. He reminded me that what I was trying to do was His job – not mine. My job was to rest in Him, to be still, to stop striving, to "let go," to surrender.

My Journal – December 16, 2009

"I'm struggling with the reality that things will never be the same because James, as he once was, is gradually slipping away. Soon only the shell of who he once was will remain. Nothing is the same without him. I realize that I'm trying to hold on to the past, to run this race, to make this journey weighed down with the memories of what once was and the regret of what will never be again. It's like running and trying to reach the goal line but never getting there because of the heavy weight I'm carrying. My "backpack" is much too heavy. It is slowing me down and sometimes I'm so exhausted, I want to give up. That's where I've been for the past week.

God is showing me, in my quiet time with Him, that I will never finish this race and reach the prize He has for me until I lay down, at His feet, my burden of grief over what is lost. With His revelation, today I am surrendering the past, and all that once was, to Him. I'm praying and asking Him to help me look ahead, not back at the way things were. With His help, I will "let go" and concentrate on where I am going in this "new normal," the future He has planned for James and me. As I pray, God's Spirit is assuring me that He has an incredible "future" for us and that He will always be with us in that future. I am greatly strengthened and encouraged by his promises and His love."
(Lucy)

e. Maybe it was because James was so sweet and
ng faith in God and His ability to meet our needs

reason, not having a connection with other
ating my new world of caregiving more difficult.

m sharing with you, as one caregiver to another, the
during our thirteen-year journey with Alzheimer's.
you to reach out for the resources that are now
rs:

eimer's Association

RP Caregiving Resource Center

th CarePartners in Houston, Texas

Care.com

kheit, CEO and Founder of AgingCare.com, states
t resource was born from a family discussion about the
sharing caregiving experiences with one another. This
ting place where caregivers can go to gain knowledge,
rength by connecting with others who are sharing similar
To quote Mr. Burkheit). It also provides articles, forums,
d questions – all moderated by care-giving experts.

ear, in the spring of 2014, the first AgingCare.com magazine
press. I discovered Vol. 1, Spring 2014 at my doctor's office.
th wonderful stories of fellow caregivers. I was thrilled when
wealth of information available. One of my favorite personal
that of Amy Grant, who has won the title of best-selling
ry Christian music performer in history. She shares her story
nts' dementia, and of her and her sisters' roles in their care. I
ote her insights concerning caregiving: "At some point in life
that some things really matter and some things don't. Living
elebrating life matters. Seeing the value in hard time's matters.
hips matter. Faith matters."

There will be times on our journey when we feel that life can never again make sense; can never again offer hope. There will be times when we reach a point where we feel helpless and alone – where we can't see anything good ahead. These are the times when all we can do is trust and surrender our hopelessness and helplessness to God the Father. At this point, all we need to do is "show up" and ask God to put back together the broken pieces of our lives. When we do, we find Him right there, right in the middle of our pain. Right where we are.

When we realize that God never allows pain without purpose, we will be ready to accept what we do not understand.

James' "life verse" and now mine, is Proverbs 3:5-6. You will probably find this verse scattered throughout this book, but its message never gets old. I'm quoting from *The Message*: "Trust God from the bottom of your heart; don't try to figure out everything on your own. Listen to God's voice in everything you do, everywhere you go; He's the one who will keep you on track." What Solomon is telling us in this verse is, don't try to understand everything. We don't need to, even if we could.

When we finally abandon and let go of the idea that we can do anything without God's help, then we will see just how "able" He really is to keep us just where we need to be – on track. And, we can rest. "Thank You, Father."

One precious husband, his memory robbed by
Alzheimer's, but his spirit safe with God.
God's gift to me.

One broken, lonely heart surrendered to God,
The Mender-of-Broken Hearts.
This, God, my gift to Thee.
~Lucy

What God's Call to Surrender Means

1. Laying all on His altar:

   My pride,

   My strengths and weaknesses,

   My perfectionism,

   My time,

   My gifts and talents.

2. Admitting that I can't "fix" everything. That's not my responsibility – it's Gods.

3. Stepping away from despair and discouragement

4. Shaping my worries into prayers

5. Surrendering all my anxieties and doubts to Him

6. Surrendering daily to God's plans for me.

"For I know the plans I have for you," declares the
Lord, "plans to prosper you and not to harm you, plans
to give you hope and a future"
(Jeremiah 29:11).

We can all agree t
of a caregiver. B
of the most rewarding a
for me as I cared for my
of somehow giving back
before Alzheimer's gradua.

The old saying, "
because it's somehow comfo
is not unique. Millions of ot
debilitating illnesses. Statistic
68 seconds someone in Ameri
us that family caregivers provid
annually.

Former first lady Rosalyn
tion: "There are only four kinds o
been caregivers; those who currer
caregivers; and those who will need

All of these statistics and ot
most troubling thing about this is tl
time when their loved one will need
is involved, what questions to ask, or
certainly didn't.

It didn't take long for me to discov
frustrating and always overwhelming. As
physical stress took a toll on me, and I
Looking back I'm not sure why I didn't
available to me. Maybe it was because I'm

9   November 2012, aarp.org/bulletin, p.

of counseling experienc
loving. I'm sure my str
was a primary factor.

Whatever the
caregivers made navig

This is why I'
lessons I've learned
I strongly encourag
available to caregive

The Alzh

The AA

Interfa

Aging

Joe Bud
that this Intern
importance of
created "a me
comfort and st
experiences" (
discussions, a

This
came off the
It is filled wi
I found the
stories was
contempor
of her pare
want to q
you realiz
matters. (
Relations

The following is an excerpt taken from *Your Name is Hughes Hannable Shanks: A Caregivers Guide to Alzheimer's, which* is a personal account of Lela Shank's years as caregiver to her husband with AD. She became an expert by reading everything she could find on AD.

Electronics for AD Patients

One day I thought, "There must be a way to use this advanced technology to help us with our loved ones." I decided to experiment. I recorded on an audio tape a 20-minute history of my husband's life, talking directly to him. I started out saying, your name is…you live at… your phone number is… you live with me, Lela, your wife, at…(again repeating our address.)" Then I continued with a brief life history, telling all the wonderful things he has done – actually praising him and building him up. (Everything I say is true, too.) I repeat his full name and address several times.

He loves the tape. I play it every morning before he gets out of bed. Every time he hears the tape, it is the first time. He smiles, sometimes tearing up, but always seems to have a good feeling from hearing it. He usually asks me, "How did 'she' know all that about me?" (Not knowing who I am.)

I told our four children about the success with the audio tape, and two of them who live in other states made videotapes of their families for Hughes. They speak directly to him with the camera zooming in on their faces. They wave to him, take him on a tour of their homes and say several times, "Hi, daddy. I love you." He smiles and waves back. He perks up when our daughter-in-law or son-in-law call out his name, Hughes. (He probably remembers that better than anything.) He usually thinks our children are his older sister and brother. More importantly, he appears to get a sense of well-being and security. I use the video tapes like a sitter if I have to run an errand. My next project is to videotape him while he can still laugh and walk and function.

~Lela Shanks
10/4/88

Caregiver's Bill of Rights

You must survive, and you have the right to.

Sometimes you need a few hours away from you're impaired loved one, and you deserve it.

You have the right to go off and find yourself again in some personal pursuit, and you need to.

You have the right to get help. You are not indispensable; let others act in your place.

You have the right to be patient with yourself and your limitations; all you can do is all you can do.

It is an important job to be caregiver for another person; it is just as important to care for you too.

Guidance for the Journey

1. Admit your fallibility and limitations. We are not Superman or Wonder Woman. We are flawed people who are coping with the assaults that life sometimes brings. Develop a sense of humor and learn to laugh about not being perfect.

2. Discuss with your loved one your feelings of uncertainty, dread, and grief. Communication and honesty are keys to healthy coping. Challenges can be met more easily together than alone.[10]

Ode to My Caregiver

Do not ask me to remember.
Don't try to make me understand.
Let me rest and know you're with me.
Kiss my cheek and hold my hand.

I'm confused beyond your concept.
I am sad and sick and lost.
All I know is that I need you
To be with me at all cost.

Do not lose your patience with me.
Do not scold or curse or cry.
I can't help the way I'm acting,
Can't be different though I try.

Just remember that I need you,
That the best of me is gone.
Please don't fail to stand beside me,
Love me till my life is done.

Author Unknown

---

10   Author's notes, Interfaith CarePartners, Roller Coaster Emotions by Earl E. Shelp, Ph.D., Conference, 2011.

Chapter 12

God's Provisions from A to Z

One of the best parts of a trip, for me, has always been the planning, the preparation, and the packing. I am meticulous about packing, trying to anticipate everything I will need for each day. Also, I allow for unforeseen emergencies, which means that I end up taking more than is necessary. I work from a carefully prepared list that, by the time I leave, has been checked and rechecked.

This trip into the unknown territory of Alzheimer's was different. I had no idea where this road would lead, what James and I would need for our journey, or how long the journey would last. Thankfully, God our faithful Guide knew. He has always known, even before we were conceived, that we would be starting this journey with Alzheimer's. He had already begun planning, preparing, and packing into His Word and into our hearts everything He knew we would need. He had already carefully and meticulously planned for all the days ahead. Whew. What a relief.

Each day I'm discovering more and more about God – that he is always anticipating our needs. He is always on time. He delivers what we need – not too early, not too late, but just at the right moment. I'm also discovering that He is providing much more than just the necessities. He is blessing us with an abundance, just as He promised. God the Son said, "I am the Good Shepherd… "I came that they may have and enjoy life, and have it in abundance, (to the full, till it overflows") (John 10:10 *AMP*).

When I began thinking of all the provisions that God had planned, prepared and packed for our journey, I began documenting them. I was amazed. I realized how many blessings I had, until then, taken for granted.

My Journal — August 15, 2008

"As I've been thinking about this chapter about God's provisions for our journey, I took a break and went to my local Walgreens. James loves to go there, and it is a nice outing for him. Since school is starting in a few days, the aisles were flooded with loving, if somewhat overwhelmed, parents holding school supply lists. They were accompanied by all sizes of eager offspring. The small ones are thrilled with the prospects of new crayons. They, of course, want the largest box available, regardless of what the list says.

I'm sure that department stores and shoe stores are also doing booming" business at the start of this new school year. Almost all parents are concerned that their children have the very best that they can afford. Many will sacrifice so that their children will have what they need, and even a little more. Just one new special outfit, cool shoes, and an awesome backpack for the first day of school can make a tremendous difference to a student, especially to a teenager. I know this because I have two fifteen-year-old grandsons with whom I spend time. I've already checked with them (and their younger brothers) to be sure they have everything they need to begin this new year with confidence.

If earthly parents (and grandparents) are so concerned about their children's needs, how much greater is our Heavenly Father's concern for His children's needs. God the Father is more keenly aware of our needs than we are. He has our supply list in His hand at all times. He will never let us do without His best for us. After all, He has an unlimited supply of everything on our "list."

We are like the first-graders in the store who are dependent on their parents to purchase what they need to be adequately equipped for school. We too are entirely dependent on God for our supply of His grace needed for our lives each day.

"Thank You, Father, that we can face each day confident that You will supply all that we need."(Lucy)

❧

Your heart may be so broken, your dreams so shattered, your needs so great, you may be wondering if anything or anyone can help. I want you to know that God can and will heal your broken heart, give you new dreams, and meet your every need. As you travel your journey with Alzheimer's, you will find that He has provided everything you need – from "A" to "Z."

Come—and See.

~ Angels ~

On our journey with Alzheimer's we will experience countless anxious moments, adverse circumstances, and agonizing loss. Although God is not the author of these things, He knows that we live in a broken world, and He will provide all that we need to overcome whatever happens on our journey.

One of God's provisions is the presence and help of angels, something we will need far more than we may ever realize.

Do you believe in angels? We all have mental pictures of angels: charming little cherubs with sweet faces, wings, and halos, dressed in gauzy white robes. Or, maybe you imagine tall, muscular figures with long white robes, mighty wings and incredibly wise and glowing countenances. Maybe your mental picture is of a muscular figure in a helmet and shiny armor.

Every Christian should be encouraged and strengthened by these truths: angels are real; angels are watching; angels mark our path. They oversee the events of our lives, always at work to promote God's plan and to bring about God's highest will for us. Their existence is mentioned almost three hundred times in the Bible. Their numbers run into the millions – ten thousand times ten thousand (Revelation 5:11).

I am deeply grateful that we are the subjects of their individual concerns, although we may not be aware of their presence. Psalm 34:7 tells us, "The angel of the Lord encamps around those who fear him and he delivers them." Eugene Peterson's *The Message,* reads, "God's angel sets up a circle of protection around us while we pray."

Angels have always played a profound role in the lives of God's people. Throughout the Bible are examples of how God used them to make His will known and to communicate His decisions to men—men such as Abraham, Moses and Jacob. Angels were also a part of the exodus of God's people out of Egypt. Numbers 20:16 reads, "When we cried out to the Lord, he heard our cry and sent an angel and brought us out of Egypt.

Joshua 5:13-15 tells us that when Joshua was near Jericho, he looked up to see a man standing in front of him with a sword in his hand. When Joshua asked him, "Are you for us or our enemies?" the man replied, "Neither, but as commander of the army of the Lord, I have now come."

Of course, one of our favorite angel stories is recorded in the book of Luke. It is the story of the Angel Gabriel appearing to Mary and telling her that she has been chosen to be the mother of Jesus, the long awaited Messiah.

All of these stories give me "goose bumps." But you may be asking, "What does all of this mean to me today? How does it affect me and my circumstances?" Well, for starters, we must believe the truth that God is the same yesterday, today and forever. When we believe that, we can believe that He is still capable of sending angels into the midst of our everyday lives to meet our needs. Not every circumstance in our lives requires an angel, but just knowing that one is standing by is very comforting to me.

I can recall at least two times in the past when, in critical danger, I was warned by an unseen presence, and my life was spared. The first incident took place when I was a child. I was visiting my grandmother, my Mamaw, on her farm. I was playing in the sand beside a small, dry creek bed near the house. I was laying on my stomach, building corrals for doodle bugs with small rocks. Suddenly I heard a rustling sound that made me raise my head. I found myself looking into the eyes of a large snake. Since I am dreadfully afraid of snakes, my first instinct was to scream and run. Just then, I heard an authoritative voice saying, "Lucy, don't move." I instantly obeyed, and within seconds the snake turned and slithered out of sight.

Even as a child, I recognized that God had protected me. When I ran to tell my Mamaw what had happened, she reached for me and held me tight, tears in her eyes. She said that the snake, according to my description, was probably a Copperhead, a very deadly snake. She said, "Surely an angel of the Lord was watching over you while you played." I remember this experience as if it were yesterday instead of seventy years ago. That experience encourages me even today as I must rely more and more on God for help and protection.

Another incident occurred about twenty-five years ago when, as a School Nurse, I was making home visits. There was a railroad track near my school that I frequently crossed to get to many of my families. That day, I approached the intersection where I would need to turn left after crossing the tracks. When the left-turn traffic light turned green, I was almost on the tracks when I heard a very loud voice in my left ear, "Lucy, stop." I looked to my left to see a train approaching, its whistle now blowing. I stomped on the brake and stopped just in time; the train barely missed me as it passed. No one could explain why the traffic lights were still working instead of blinking as they should have been or why the crossing arms were not down. But I do know this. God had placed an angel in my car that day to protect me and to deliver me from harm.

To this very day, I never get behind the wheel of my car without asking God to surround me with angels. Then I thank Him for his protection for me and the other drivers on the streets.

As James' Alzheimer's advanced, I often found myself afraid during the night. James had always been so strong and confident, almost over-protective of me. I was never afraid of anything when I was with him. During this time in 2001, in our wonderful new neighborhood, there had been a home invasion. Now, I was not only afraid for myself but for James. I knew that in the event of any danger – fire, storm, home invasion or break-in – I would be responsible, not just for myself, but for him as well. Especially for him.

In the midst of this, my "uneasy season", "9/11" occurred. Now the whole nation was fearful, even those with a strong faith in God. We had seen the cruel face of the enemy. A week after this terrorist attack on our country, I had a terrifying dream. In the dream, James and I were sleeping when I was suddenly awakened. I looked through our bedroom door and down the hall. I saw two or three armed men, closely resembling those we had seen portrayed on television as being the terrorists. They were entering one of the bedrooms that opened into the hall. I slipped out of bed and woke James, trying to get him up and into a "safe room" off our master bedroom. He didn't want to go, and he broke away from me to go down the hall where there were the men with guns. I ran to safety, knowing with certainty what would happen to James. I couldn't save him.

I awoke in a cold sweat. I had never been more frightened in my entire life. My heart was pounding so hard I couldn't breathe. I looked over at James, sleeping peacefully. At that moment, I realized how very fragile he is and how incapable I am, in my strength, to protect him. I began praying, asking God's forgiveness for being such a coward in my dream. I surrendered my fears to Him and asked Him for divine protection for James and me. Even then, I wondered if I would ever be able to sleep again. As I lay there, still filled with dread from my dream, I sensed a presence in our bedroom. There seemed to be soft light coming from the corner across from our bed. At that moment, the dread in my heart was replaced by peace I could not explain. I fell into a deep, restful sleep. The next morning, I realized that God must have placed an angel in our room that night. For the next twelve years, anytime I had a frightening dream or felt afraid during the night, I talked to God about it. Inevitably, I experienced that same peace, and I knew that angels were nearby.

I am aware that all this may seem too simplistic, too unrealistic, and too improbable for some of you. I also know, however, that there will be times in your life as caregiver to your loved one when you will be afraid. Times when you will need supernatural help. Remember, God specializes in the supernatural; in fact, He invented it. Just knowing that this help is available at all times, often through angels, should be a great comfort to you. It is to me.

Someone pointed out to me recently that when we get to Heaven, we will meet the angels who were assigned to help us and protect us while we were here on earth. The Scriptures tell us, in Hebrews 12:22, "You have come to Mount Zion, to the heavenly Jerusalem, the city of the living God. You have come to thousands upon thousands of angels in joyful assembly."

I wonder if I will recognize some of them, my special assigned Guardian Angels. I can't wait to hear them telling about the times they rode in the car with James and me to the VA Hospital, went to surgery with me, went to the cemetery with me, protected me on dark or dangerous streets.

Speaking of dangerous streets reminds me of the day I had jury duty in downtown Houston, Texas. I could not find a parking place near the courthouse. Rather than risking being late, I parked several blocks away. As I started walking, keeping my destination in sight, I realized I was not in an ideal part of town to be walking alone. Feeling very vulnerable, I tried not to look at the "homeless" men lining the sidewalks on either side of me. I walked very fast down the middle of the street and held my purse as close to my body as possible. Within seconds, I realized that someone was following me. Dreading what I would see, I looked over my shoulder to see a young man, dancing along, whistling and snapping his fingers. With a big smile, he said, "I gotcha back." He followed me to within a few steps of the courthouse. When I turned to thank him, there was no one there. I asked the Police Officer at the door if he had seen where the man who was following me had gone. He looked puzzled and said that there was no one following me. When I told him where I had parked and why, he said, "Don't ever do that again.

And, when you get ready to leave today, find me or another policeman to take you back to your car. That is a dangerous part of town."

In heaven, I especially want to meet again "this angel" who protected me on a dangerous Houston street. I also want to meet the angels who called my name and saved me from the snake and the train.

I believe that we will all be very surprised when we recognize some of our angels who were visible to us while here on earth. I think we will be delighted when we meet the angels we have "entertained" and aided in some way. There is a scripture that tells us to: "Keep on loving one another as brothers and sisters. Do not forget to show hospitality to strangers, for by so doing, some have shown hospitality to angels without even knowing it" (Hebrews 13:1-2). This scripture was always fascinating to me, even as a child. My paternal grandmother was a wonderful Christian and a marvelous cook. Because she lived near a railroad track, hobos often stopped at her back door for a handout. Her reputation as a generous woman and an excellent cook was shared by those riding the boxcars during the Depression when jobs and food were scarce. Grandmother never turned anyone away when they were hungry. I can remember that she made it a practice to prepare extra biscuits and sausage every morning. I can also remember sitting on the back steps beside total strangers who didn't smell like soap and water, eating my biscuit with them. This demonstration of love for strangers made a definite impression on my heart, one that remains today. When I get to heaven, I have a feeling some of those men with whom I shared a biscuit might be a part of that "joyful assembly of angels."

As strange as it may seem, as I have been polishing this chapter on angels today, August 9, 2013, I stopped to watch ABC World News with Diane Sawyer. She is telling the story of what had happened that day to a young woman. I missed some of the details, but apparently her car had been crushed in a horrible accident, and she was trapped inside. No amount of effort on the part of rescue workers could free this critically injured young woman, even though they used all the equipment available to them. The girl asked that those standing around pray aloud. Suddenly, according to witnesses, a man appeared, dressed in black like a priest and carrying a small bottle. He went to the girl, laid his hand on her and started praying loudly. Just then, a new crew of rescue workers arrived with just the right equipment needed to free the girl from her car. After she was freed and taken away by ambulance, no one could find the man in black who had prayed for her. Although dozens of pictures were taken at the scene by many photographers, the man was not in any of the photos. The news program ended with Diane Sawyer asking the question, "Was the man in black an angel?"

I certainly have no problem believing that he was. However, in the often skeptical, high-tech society in which we live today, many consider things like angels and miracles mere myths, fairy tales too good to be true. These skeptics are missing out on many of God's blessings and provisions because of their unbelief. Not only has God provided the greatest Gift, everlasting life through faith in His Son, Jesus, He has provided everything else we need, including an Angel Army.

Maybe you have an angel story to tell. If so, tell your story. It may be the very thing that will encourage others on their journey. I pray that my stories have encouraged you, fellow caregiver. I'll be thanking God for His provision of ministering angels who watch over us and who are aware of all the details of our earthly journey. We must never forget who is in the heavenly grandstands keeping a close eye on us, cheering us on to victory.

~ Beauty ~

Beauty is a gift from God that is important to all of us. It is, however, sometimes difficult to define because it means different things to different people. No matter how we explain it, beauty satisfies within us a longing for something to dispel the blandness, the ugliness, the darkness, the despair in our lives. Alzheimer's caregivers can certainly identify with that statement. Some forces in our lives are very powerful. Examples are the endless tasks of caregiving: the exhaustion, the discouragement, the loneliness, the drudgery. These things can blind us to the reality that beauty does exist and that it is a gift from God.

Beloved Caregiver, we have a beautiful Heavenly Father who has packed this provision of beauty for us to enjoy. Psalm 27:4 states:

"One thing I ask of the Lord, this is

what I seek: that I may dwell in the

house of the Lord all the days of my

life, to gaze upon the beauty of

the Lord and to seek Him in

His temple."

Sometimes in the midst of the daily drudgery of caring for our loved one with dementia, we forget to look for the beauty around us. Perhaps your heart is too heavy to look up and see God revealed in the trees and flowers and the sky. All of nature sings His praise, but we must make the effort to hear and to lift our eyes to experience His divine nature revealed through His creation. Perhaps you, like I, can no longer travel, can no longer take those wonderful trips to the mountains or the ocean, or to the Texas bluebonnet fields in the Spring with your loved one. Perhaps you were too tired this year to plant flowers or to maintain those already growing in your yard or planters. Perhaps you, like I, have given up your home, your yard, your garden to move to a more appropriate place where you can receive needed help.

When, in obedience to God's instructions, I sold our beautiful "miracle house" on Rainbow Bend, I felt empty, depleted, barren. It was my "blue, white, and yellow" dream house filled with all the beautiful things I had so lovingly collected through the years. My blue and white teapots and china, the blue and white French toile curtains I had painstakingly made for the living room and dining room. The big pine hutch filled with my mother's Blue Willow dishes and my Mamaw's antique platters.

By the time I had staged and cleaned our home for showing, I was exhausted, physically and emotionally. Thankfully, God graciously and miraculously, on April 1, 2010, sold the house fifteen minutes after the "For Sale" sign went up. The first couple who saw it loved it – (who wouldn't?) That was the one thing I had asked God for – that the first person who saw it would love it, would be happy with the asking price, and would buy it.

Within a month, with the help of my wonderful children and friends, I had sold, given away and thrown away much of my fifty-three years of collection of "things." James and I were moving from our large house to a two-room apartment at a Brookdale Assisted Living Community, the Hampton, in Pearland, Texas. This special two-room apartment had been created just for us. Next door to our building was the Memory Care facility, Clare Bridge, where James would be spending eight or nine hours each day.

By the time all the papers were signed, and we were no longer Homeowners for the first time in over fifty years, I was more than ready to accept all the help available to us. For the past two years, James and I had been primarily homebound, and I was looking forward to going back to church, getting together with friends, and just resting.

Living at the Hampton was like living in a hotel. Our apartment was lovely. It was filled with the blue, yellow, and white material things I loved the most. There was no clutter. (No room for clutter.) I had a precious cleaning lady who kept our two rooms sparkling. We had maintenance men to take care of any technical needs. Across the hall was an exercise room leading out onto a beautiful deck. Each morning one of the Care Associates from our building walked James next door to Clare Bridge for the day. Then in the evening a Care Associate from there walked him back to our apartment. Oh, I almost forgot one of the best things: three times a day, I went downstairs to a beautiful dining room where I was served excellent meals.

This may sound like Heaven to those of you who are caring for your loved one at home. However, leaving my house, my neighbors, and the church that we attended, which I could see from my front door, was more painful than I can put into words. I knew this was God's plan, but I grieved for what would no longer be.

I was so exhausted the first few weeks I just wanted to rest. I missed my "Bethel" in my previous home, but I still had my blue chair, and I quickly established a new Bethel where I spent uninterrupted hours with the Lord and His Word. After breakfast, after James was safely and – I must add – happily next door, I immersed myself and my wounded heart in quiet times of worship and prayer.

There came a time when the enormity of the change, the reality of my drastic New Normal began to sink in. Then I went through a period of grief. Sometimes when I was so lonely, even while surrounded by people, I would go out onto the upstairs deck across from my apartment.

My Journal — June 2, 2010
(One month after we moved in.)

"Father, today I feel lost and lonely. Nothing seems familiar, and I'm wondering where I am and how I got here. I am outside on the deck, looking out over the beautifully kept grounds.

Thank you, Father, for this beautiful place with its green lawns, trees, shrubs, and beautiful flower beds everywhere. I look up and see an unobstructed expanse of sky. This morning, as I look up at the sky, I have a strong sense that You are there, watching me from on high. The sky you have created is always amazing. Today, the sky is a blue sea with a few puffy, white cloud islands. The unblemished blue of the sky is so beautiful it takes my breath away and brings tears to my eyes. And I am comforted by this beauty and Your presence."(Lucy)

My Journal — August 31, 2010

This morning when I went out on the deck, the sky was a huge gray canopy filled with dark clouds that twirled and danced across the horizon, occasionally chased by flashes of lightening. I think my favorite is the sky at dawn, just as the first rays of the sun peep over the eastern horizon, heralding the new day and dispelling the darkness of the night and my spirit. I go out early only when James is still sleeping soundly, and I can safely slip away long enough to greet the day and experience the breathtaking beauty of the sunrise. Our upstairs apartment is on the west side of our building and each evening I can watch unobstructed, gorgeous sunsets from my windows. Each time, I think about how blessed I am to have a ringside seat to such beauty. Watching the last tiny slice of red sun slip over the edge of the earth is something I had never before been privileged to experience. I am so touched by God's goodness, and each breath-taking sunset brings me closer to the Creator of such wonder and beauty. (Lucy)

After James' death, I have remained in the house I had built in 2011. It's a beautiful house just around the comer, 30 seconds from Clare Bridge where James lived full time for his last year. My primary goal and purpose during this season is to complete the book I began writing in 2008. I have tried to keep from making any commitments until the book is finished. I feel that this is my ministry for now, as my body and heart are recovering from my thirteen-year journey. Writing about the past is not always easy, but it is still therapeutic just as it was at the beginning of this journey.

My Journal – November 1, 2012

Today as I was rewriting and editing this chapter about God's gift of Beauty, I turned on my television to a program with soothing background music and wonderful nature scapes. Today's subject is "mountains of Western America." As I watched, I was transported back in time to the wonderful vacations James and I took to New Mexico, Colorado, and Wyoming. Mountains have always thrilled me like nothing else in all of God's creation. Fascinated by the beauty and the unbelievable scenes of familiar mountain ranges and passes, I was moved to put into words the emotions I was experiencing at the time. This is my offering:

A Psalm to the Creator

You, O Holy Architect, who drew the blueprints
and designed the mountains that majestically
display Your greatness,
Design something beautiful in me.
You, who carved great Cathedrals from mountain
rock and walls formed of ancient stone, standing
tall and proud on the horizon,
Form something beautiful in me.

You, who made rock monuments bravely standing
in honor of their creator, their peaks reaching the
clouds, which You formed from nothing,
Create something beautiful in me.
You, who stacked enormous rocks on top of one
another like children's building blocks, touching
the floor of Heaven,
Put together something beautiful in me.
You, the Creator and Gardener of Earth, who year
after year planted the Aspens whose leaves dance
like gold coins in the Fall breezes,
Plant something beautiful in me.
~Lucy

~ Blessings ~

On my journey with Alzheimer's, there have been many days when God has lifted me from a pit of despair and taken me to the "high places" of blessing in Him.

In Ephesians 1:3-6, in Eugene Peterson's, *The Message*, we find these wonderful words: "How blessed is God. And what a blessing He is. He's the Father of our Master, Jesus Christ and takes us to the high places of blessing in him. Long before he laid down earth's foundations, he had us in mind, had settled on us as the focus of his love, to be made whole and holy by his love. Long, long ago he decided to adopt us into his family through Jesus Christ. (What pleasure he took in planning this.) He wanted us to enter into the celebration of his lavish gift-giving by the hand of his beloved Son."

God the Father is telling each of us that, even before He created the world, we were on His mind, the focus of His love. He decided to adopt us, through our faith in Jesus Christ, to share His lavish gifts. This plan gave Him great pleasure and provided us with great blessings. How awesome is that.

Our Father, who had us in mind before time began, knows exactly what we're facing each day as we care for our loved one. He knows when we are experiencing discouragement and heartache. He wants us to know that He is blessing us and reaching down to dispense His incredible love and grace in the midst of our pain. Although His blessing may be hard to recognize through our tears and during our long, sleepless nights, we can keep trusting that He is working for us. It has been during those times that I have discovered that He truly is the God who loves me and who is always lavishing blessings on me.

"Next time a sunrise steals your breath or a meadow of flowers leaves you speechless, remain that way. Say nothing, and listen as Heaven whispers, *"Do you like it? I did it just for you."* [11]

My Journal — Thanksgiving 2009

"As I'm writing tonight about blessings, our family has just celebrated Thanksgiving Day together. Each year as we come together as a family, we are reminded that we are abundantly blessed. This year as we gather around the table, there is one thing conspicuously missing: the "Spiritual giant" of our family. James, our beloved husband, father, and Papaw is sleeping soundly.

We debated whether we should wake him, and then unanimously agreed to let him sleep. He was up most of the night, "looking for something." The only time he seems genuinely at peace is when he is sleeping.

I tried not to be sad, focusing instead on my blessings. I looked around the table at our three wonderful sons, two beautiful daughters-in-law, and five bright, healthy grandsons, and I was overwhelmed with gratitude and joy. My joy came from the knowledge that we are all God's children, joint heirs with Jesus Christ and that we will all be celebrating together throughout eternity. That knowledge is the greatest blessing anyone could receive.

After the meal, the men took care of the clean-up so that we "girls" could take our traditional Thanksgiving afternoon shopping trip to Garden Ridge. By now, James was up, dressed, with my help, and fed. He was settled in his recliner, watching football with the other men as I left. I kissed him and assured him that I would return soon. The report, on my return from shopping, was that

11   *Self Help Daily, Inspirational Quotes* by Author Max Lucado.

every five minutes, he would ask, "Where's Lucy? When is she coming back?" Needless to say, he was not the only one glad to see me when we returned from shopping.

Later, after the others had left to go to a movie, James and I snuggled together on the couch. I was exhausted by now. Because James had been awake most of the night, I too had slept very little. My "endless energy" and boundless strength" to get up at 5:30 in the morning to put an enormous turkey into the oven, make a huge pan of dressing, and prepare the rest of my traditional Thanksgiving meal, are tangible proofs of God's blessings. They are "the utter extravagance of His work in me" (Ephesians 1:19-20, The Message).

The shopping trip, however, had taken its toll on my feet. I realized that just being there with James, propping up my tired feet, holding his hand, I was content and at peace. As I reflected on the past year, these were some of my thoughts:

- Although there have been days this past year when I have wanted to give up, God stepped onto the mat and fought my battles for me.

- Although God has not chosen to heal James, something that I, and others, have prayed for daily, He has kept James sweet and funny and physically healthy.

- God has given me emotional and physical strength and stamina just when I needed it.

- God has given me peace in my valleys of despair. I have a new, sacred intimacy with Him.

- When I have felt alone, helpless, and depressed, He has always been there to remind me that He is my hope, my joy, and my constant companion.

I looked at these generous blessings from God, and I realized these were things we have received, not in spite of but because of the tragedy that is Alzheimer's. It is a tragedy that keeps me on my knees daily as I seek God's strength, guidance, and wisdom for the day.

As I shared these blessings with James, he said, "Thank You, Lord." Then he said, "We're so blessed. Why are we so blessed?" My answer "Because we love and trust God, who loves us and who loves to bless us." And James said, "Amen." (Lucy)

My Journal — February 17, 2012

"It's been more than two years since I began writing this chapter about blessings. God is even more dear to me today than He was back then, in November of 2009. I'm discovering daily that when we live our lives according to God's plan for us, we are blessed, and God is glorified. This morning I was reading Matthew 5:3-4 in Eugene Peterson's, "The Message." These verses, part of the Beatitudes, are Jesus' words to his disciples:

Verse 3: "You're blessed when you're at the end of your rope. With less of you, there is more of God and His rule."

Sound familiar? I don't know about you, but I have been at the "end of my rope" most of the time in these last thirteen years on our journey with Alzheimer's. "Thank You, Father, that, during these years, I have always found You waiting at the end of my rope."

Verse 4: "You're blessed when you feel you've lost what is most dear to you. Only then can you be embraced by the One most dear to you." (Lucy)

I could write an entire book about loss. In fact, that's what I'm doing. But then, the book is as much about God's precious provisions as it is about the loss. It is about my realization that He is all that I need. Would I have known this wonderful intimacy with God my Father, with Jesus and the Holy Spirit, had I not lost what is so dear to me? The loss of the beautiful life James and I shared, the special intimacy, companionship, and friendship that a great marriage provides is more painful than I could have ever imagined. But then, the blessings of the fresh, sweet presence and the joy of the Lord in my heart is more comforting than I could have imagined.

It is in the midst of my mourning that I am discovering God's special blessings for me – His comfort, His peace, His hope, His joy, His love. These blessings, poured out on me twenty-four hours a day, are precious jewels quarried from the mine of loneliness, exhaustion, and sorrow.

Today, I will celebrate His blessings by focusing on everything excellent and beautiful on my journey with Him. I will count my blessings instead of my losses, and I will be grateful for His gifts that are too numerous to count.

I was reading some thoughts in an article by Max Lucado that I hope will shine a bright light on God and all of His wonderful blessings. I'm sharing some of his words with you:

"A grateful heart sees each day as a gift. Thankful people focus less on what they lack and more on the privileges they have. I attended a banquet recently in which a wounded soldier was presented with the gift of a free house. He nearly fell over with gratitude. He bounded onto the stage with his one good leg and threw both arms around the presenter. 'Thank you. Thank you. Thank you.' He hugged the guitar player in the band and the big woman on the front row. He thanked the waiter, the other soldiers, and then the presenter again. Before the night was over, he thanked me. And I didn't do anything. Shouldn't we be equally grateful? Jesus is building a house for us (John 14:2). Our deed of ownership is every bit as certain as that of the soldier." [12]

12   *Attitude of Gratitude: Be Thankful*, Devotional by Max Lucado at http://thoughts-about-god.com/blog/2014/10/13/ml_an-attitude-of-gratitude.

I'm concluding this chapter with some feelings about a song played frequently on Christian radio station KSBJ, during the year 2012. So many times, it would be playing as I made my three-times-a-day trip from my house to Clare Bridge where James lived from October 1, 2011 until his death, September 17, 2012. I would sit in the car in front of his building until the song ended. Each time I felt that it was a gift from God to me. The song was sung at James' funeral. The words may not have been meaningful to everyone in our packed church, but they were to me. The song is *Blessings* by Laura Story, from the album, *Blessings*. Laura's sweet, plaintive voice and the hauntingly beautiful music and lyrics always ministered to me in the midst of my heartaches. Laura wrote it during the five years she struggled with her young husband's brain tumor and the after effects of it. She learned and passed on several lessons expressed in the lyrics. For me the most important lesson is that blessings from God don't always come in the perfect packages we expect. The words of this song helped me realize that the trials, storms, tears, and thousands of sleepless nights may be sent by God to draw us closer to Himself and to reveal to us that this is not our home. As James would say, "It's not our real home."

~ Burden Bearer ~

"Pile your troubles on God's Shoulders – He'll carry your load,
He'll help you out" (Psalm 55:23 *The Message*).

Beloved Caregiver, aren't you glad that we have a Burden-Bearer whose shoulders are wide enough to carry our heavy burdens on our journey into the unknown of Alzheimer's. God has promised in His Word to do this for us. When we surrender our cares and burdens to Him, they are no longer ours. They now belong to Him. What an incredible truth.

"We often marvel at someone who has done a particular feat daily for years and years. I am reminded of a fellow who has run every day since the early 1910s. Truly remarkable when you think how life often attempts and succeeds to derail our daily plans. There is something to be said for faithfulness and perseverance of this sort.

Is there ever a day that you know you should do something, yet you blow it off? We have all done this. However, God never tires of daily bearing our burden. If all 6 billion souls on this planet turned to Jesus this very day, He would still be strong enough to carry every care and woe of the human race. All we must do is trust, surrender and rely upon Him as the "God, who is our salvation."[13]

My Journal — January 5, 2008

"My memories of life without the constant burden of Alzheimer's are growing dimmer day by day. It's getting steadily harder to remember when my heart, my spirit, and my body were not bent over under this constant burden of caregiving. Only those who have experienced it can truly understand the exhaustion of being responsible for a loved one twenty-four hours a day, seven days a week. Today, I am still dealing with the problems caused by an overflowing commode in our master bathroom. This happened the middle of December, during the week of the Singing Christmas Tree. Thankfully I was miraculously at home between performances (The complete story is in the chapter on "Wisdom"). It was God's loving way of letting me know that I could never again leave James home alone. All the cleanup and repairs were an inconvenience while trying to get ready for the holidays, but now everything is finished except the new carpet for our Master closet. God is so faithful." (Lucy)

My Journal — January 15, 2008

"Our new lifestyle description, "Homebound," is almost as depressing as it sounds. Already, I am finding myself drifting further from my support system — my church, my

---

13   The Bare Soul Daily Devotional, Our Burden Bearer, by Rick Roeber, Thursday, January 17, 2013.

friends, my family. People are so busy, sometimes I think that they forget I'm here. Loneliness, however, is a regular visitor. Although my precious James, the love of my life, is here, he is gradually becoming almost a shell of the bright, productive man he once was. I listen to the sound of his shuffling feet as he wanders through a house that has become unfamiliar to him. His endless, repetitive questions make up our conversations. Depression has come to the door recently but it is an uninvited, unwelcome burden, and I hurry to roll it over onto Jesus' shoulders. I know carrying it on my shoulders can cause pain and other health problems. I try to stay focused on maintaining my amazing, supernatural health and energy – a gift from God the Father." (Lucy)

My Journal — Father's Day Weekend, June 2009

Our sons and their families were all here this weekend to spend Father's Day with James. When our son and daughter-in-law from San Antonio arrived, they were very concerned about my health. They said they could see my exhaustion and stress reflected in my eyes, the dark circles a dead giveaway. They could see it in the way my clothes are beginning to hang loosely on my weary body. I don't want the children to worry about me. We all sat down and discussed my options. There are no easy answers at this point. The children know that I am trusting God to take care of their Dad and me and that I am always asking for divine wisdom.

We discussed the possibility of hiring sitters or trying to find an Alzheimer's Day Care facility. Both of these options have negative and positive features. We didn't reach any decisions, but we all agreed to pray for God's perfect answer and solution for our situation. I know that God has a plan that He will reveal at just the right time. I will wait for Him."
(Lucy)

I know the One who has promised to bear our burdens for us. It's just that it's so difficult at times to fully trust this promise because we don't know exactly what it looks like translated into our real life situations. I'm not worried, however. I know that when I pray, "I need You, Father. Please help me.", He will always answer, and I am never disappointed.

The following is an Ad one might see in the "Help Wanted" section of my weary heart:

HELP WANTED

Alzheimer's Caregiving:
A Load too Heavy
Needed: A Burden Bearer
for a Safari into the Unknown.
~Lucy

I know that my Heavenly Father will answer this "ad," this prayer, immediately after I "place" it. The word "safari" reminds me of Africa. It is a continent I have loved since childhood when I sang, "Jesus loves the little children of the world." As I sang the words, I too fell in love with the African children, a love that remains today. As long as I can remember, I have watched almost every movie made about Africa, filmed in Africa. As a child watching "Tarzan" movies, I was fascinated by the bearers, young African men who carried on their heads and backs the heavy supplies for the hunters and explorers. I marveled at their strength, agility, sure-footedness, and courage. They never seemed to worry about snakes or other dangers. They were focused and committed to those they served. At the end of each day's long journey, they set up camp, cooked, served and cleaned up. At night, they kept watch, protecting against wild animals. They never seemed to be tired; they never sat idle, doing nothing.

Like these bearers, our Burden Bearer never sleeps, never slumbers, is never tired, never turns His cell phone off. He is always available, day or night, to serve us and to protect us. I love Psalms 121: 1-4. It tells me that my help comes from the Lord, who will not let me fall. "He who watches over you will not slumber; indeed, he who watches over Israel will neither slumber nor sleep." Verses seven and eight tell us, "the Lord will keep you from all harm—he will watch over your life; the Lord will watch over your coming and going both now and forevermore."

With promises like these, why would we ever worry? It is only when we are exhausted and our "defenses are down" that Satan whispers discouragement into our minds. I want to walk in complete dependence on God, my faithful Burden-Bearer. Sometimes, however, at the end of the day, I feel worn out, frazzled and depleted. This long, exhausting Season would be a hopeless narrative of my life as James' full-time caregiver were it not for the relentless faithfulness of the One who has promised to bear my burdens.

Each morning at my "Bethel", I lay my heavy burden of long days and sleepless nights at His feet. I surrender my loneliness and depression, my fears and frustrations, my worries and anxieties, my weakness and exhaustion, my helplessness and hopelessness. I open my Bible to a marked scripture that is underlined, highlighted and dated: "Praise be to the Lord, to God our Savior who daily bears our burdens" (Psalm 68:19).

Then, I exchange my loneliness and depression for His comfort and joy, my fears and frustrations for His courage, my worries and anxieties for His peace, my weakness and exhaustion for His strength, my helplessness and hopelessness for His hope.

When in faith and trust I surrender my load of cares to my Father, the perfect Burden-Bearer, I can begin the day ahead with renewed strength and "peace that passes understanding." Today I will ask God my Father, the Lifter-of-my head, to renew, refresh and remind me that eventually He will restore all that I have lost. Knowing that He is walking beside me, carrying my heavy load, gives me courage for the day.

This simple story says it all: "A father stands at the window watching as his small son struggles to remove a large, heavy rock from his sandbox, with no success. After watching for a moment, the father walks out and effortlessly picks up the rock. He says, "Son, you should have called your Dad. I'm always standing by to help you."

~ Comfort ~

This chapter about God's comfort in our times of grief has been very difficult to write. There are so many things I want to share with you. I've spent two days trying to decide where to begin. I'm sharing my deepest feelings with you to let you know that grieving is okay; it's normal; it's important. Grief, if not expressed, can make one bitter and old. I don't want that to happen to you or to me.

Although grief is ugly and wrenching, it is unavoidable. It's important that we talk about it. God's provision of comfort in our times of grief is essential for our journey into a world of sadness and loss. Comfort is a loving provision from the heart of God the Father, who mourns with us as we grieve, and from God the Son, Jesus, who carried our sorrows and who is well acquainted with grief.

Grief and loss are an inevitable part of life. God gives, and He takes away. He has a reason for everything, even when the reason doesn't make sense to us. While living with Alzheimer's, we will have seasons of grief and heartache, but there will also be seasons of joy.

God's Word tells us in James 1: 2-3: "Consider it pure joy, my brothers, whenever you face trials of many kinds because you know that the testing of your faith develops perseverance."

"Come meet the God of encouragement. He loves you. He never gives up on you, especially when life is hard, because he has been there. The hand that reaches out to comfort you is a pierced one."[14]

Throughout the Bible, we are told that our Heavenly Father understands our grief. He Himself experienced the worst kind of loss – the loss of an only son. He was so grief-stricken that the earth shook, and the sky became dark with His grief. He knew, however, that joy was

14   *Meet the God of Encouragement*, published by Multnomah Books, a part of the Questar Publishing family © 1994 by Max Lucado.

coming soon. When my "sky" turns dark with my grief and loss, I will remember that God's grief turned to joy in three days. We are all still celebrating that joy. I will remember with the Psalmist that "weeping may remain for a night, but rejoicing comes in the morning," (Psalm 30:5). In that same Psalm, David added, in verse eleven, "You turned my wailing into dancing; you removed my sackcloth and clothed me with joy."

Can grief and joy actually co-exist? I never thought about it until I wrote those words from *Psalm 30*. I know that grief does exist because I experience it every day. I also know that I experience joy every day, even in the midst of my sadness. God knows that there will be many days, while caring for our loved one, that our hearts will break from loneliness and loss. He tells us in Hebrews 13:5 (*The Message*), "I'll never let you down; never walk off and leave you." Today, I will choose joy and celebrate what I have instead of grieving for what I have lost.

The day in 1999 when the doctor said the dreaded word, "Alzheimer's", our lives changed forever. As James gradually lost his mental acuity, we struggled to accept what this reality would mean. Through my struggles to cope, my "spiritual acuity" became sharper. My quiet times with the Lord grew more meaningful as I cried out to Him. I began to understand more clearly His love for me and His purpose for this "disruptive" season in our lives. As difficult as it was at times, I began to thank God for this tragedy that I prayed would never happen to James (and me). Psalm 34:1 says, "Bless the Lord at all times." I realize there are things to be thankful for: my supernatural health, James' sweet nature, a growing intimacy with my Heavenly Father.

My Journal — April 14, 2003

> *"Father, today I realize how very blessed I am to have You in my life. Knowing that You are always here comforts me in this strange "season" when I feel that my life is unraveling. Because You are my life, I will cling to You, believing that You welcome my tight embrace as I cling to You in times of desperation." (Lucy)*

With many illnesses, tragedies, or even death, one can eventually return to some semblance of his previous life. With Alzheimer's, sometimes referred to as a "Living Death", this gradual death of the mind, the reasoning, and the persona of your loved one is a daily reality. This can continue for years, leaving no room for normality, only frequent "new normals" which change like the seasons. James and I have experienced many "seasons" in the past thirteen years of our journey.

My Journal — April 2, 2004, 6:30 A.M.

"I'm clinging to you today, Father. I can't survive without Your strength and comfort. You tell me in Your Word that You "go before me and will be with me; that You will never leave me or forsake me." You tell me to not to be afraid or discouraged. This morning I am reading those very words from Deuteronomy 31:8. I know that You always keep Your promises, and I will rest in them today. I am exhausted, but You already know that. James had an upset stomach, and we were up much of the night. I wonder if increasing the dosage of his medication is causing this? As You know, he doesn't always make it to the bathroom in time. Thank You for the strength to do the difficult cleanups. You are here, even in times of "drudgery." I always sense your strength and help. I'm so thankful that James is sleeping peacefully so that I can spend all the time I need with You today. You always restore me and give me supernatural strength and energy. Only You, Father, can do that. I love You, and I know You love me. (Lucy)

My Journal — March 3, 2005, 10:00 P.M.

"This has been one of "those days." I'm exhausted physically, but mentally and emotionally I need to wind down and process my feelings. More than anything, I need some quiet

time with my Heavenly Father. James had an upset stomach earlier today but was better by evening. He's on a new Alzheimer's medication.

James loves to watch Bill, Sean, and Greta on Fox News at night. He doesn't watch movies or even situation comedies because he can't follow the plot. But he enjoys the News. He especially likes Greta and recognizes her when her show comes on at 9:00 P.M.

He always says, "Honey, here's Greta. Come watch her with me."—and I do. He usually goes to sleep in his recliner shortly after her show begins.

Tonight, by 9:30, he was ready to go to bed. I got him settled, carefully covering my "little man" and kissing him. He was asleep within seconds. I will join him later.

I'm now at my Bethel. To begin this "saga", I had cleaned James and our bathroom wall and floor three times by early afternoon. After the third time I was so tired and discouraged, I sat down on the bathroom floor and cried. Sitting there, surrounded by a mop, sponge, and disinfectant, I was feeling very sorry for myself. I cried and prayed.

As I prayed, Jesus "met me there." I didn't actually see Him, but I knew He was there with me. I could picture Him sitting beside me on the floor. In my spirit, I experienced His love and comfort. It was as if He was saying to me, "Whatever you are doing for James, you are doing for me." He reminded me that after James and I married when I did something for him, I would tease him and say, "I'm doing this for you and Jesus." My godly mother had taught me this sweet lesson on submission by her example in her marriage to my father (Theirs was a beautiful marriage).

As I thought about Jesus' teaching concerning this very thing, I got up from the floor, dried my eyes, blew my nose, and found my Bible. I turned to Matthew 25. There I found the highlighted, underlined words of Jesus as he taught His disciples about the end times. He reminded them that whatever they would do, after he left, to minister to those in need of help, they would be doing for Him. Standing before King Jesus in heaven someday, they would hear these words found in Matthew 25:40: "The King will reply, 'I tell you the truth, whatever you did for one of the least of these brothers of mine, you did for Me."

Wow. That was a spiritual wake-up call, a moment of truth for me. I realized that someday I want to hear Him say those words to me. Right then I made a commitment. I would remember that, from then on, when I did anything for James, who can no longer care for himself, I would be doing it for Jesus.

As I reflect on the events of this long day, I'm thinking about how much God must love me to share with me such amazing secrets straight from heaven. This knowledge wonderfully strengthens and comforts me tonight. A day that began with tears and frustration is ending with a heart filled with love and gratitude for my Comforter." (Lucy)

Hopefully, this wonderful secret God has shared with me will help you find purpose in the inevitable drudgery as you care for your loved one.

My Journal — November 9, 2006

"Today is our forty-ninth wedding anniversary. I asked James, who has been dozing in his recliner in our bedroom if he knew what day it is. He said, "I think it is Monday." I explained that it is our wedding anniversary. He said, "Isn't that wonderful." And he went back to sleep.

At that moment, I felt a "crack" in my heart. I stood there for a minute, feeling suddenly very alone. Then, I took a deep breath, tucked an afghan around James' legs, kissed the top of his head, picked up my purse, and slipped out. I went to my favorite gift shop that is about five minutes away. My friends who work there cried with me and comforted me. They helped me to select several gifts for myself. As I left, I felt better. However, nothing that money can buy can take away the heartache and loneliness I'm feeling today." (Lucy)

My Journal — November 10, 2006

"When I read my journal entry from yesterday, I realized that I need to start sharing my heartaches with friends who care about me. "Super Moms, Super Wives, Super Christians," hesitate to show their frailties to others, feeling that they must always be strong and together. Is it a pride thing?

At my Bethel this morning, God is helping me to see that being honest and transparent won't make others think that I am "weak" or faithless." Rather, it may encourage them to know that everyone at times experiences difficulties, even those with a strong faith and commitment to God. He is also reminding me that I deny my friends the opportunity to be blessed through their ministry to me. How can they reach out to me when I am lonely and wondering if anyone knows or cares where I am and what I feel unless I share my heart with them? This may be uncomfortable at first, but I know that it is the right thing to do. That is what I would want my friends to do.

Thank You, Father, for revealing this to me." (Lucy)

Have you noticed that special occasions, like Valentine's Day, Birthdays, Thanksgiving and Christmas, and for spouses, wedding anniversaries, cause the greatest heartaches? For me, they represent some of the happiest times that I have shared with James. The fact that he can't share with me the memories of these special times is one of the hardest things for me to accept about this terrible disease. I have to dig very deep into my inner strength to survive the red-letter days, especially our wedding anniversaries.

෴

My Journal — Sunday November 9, 2007

6:30 A.M. "Today is our 50th Wedding Anniversary. James and I had always talked about how we would celebrate this day. If we had daughters, we knew they would probably want to plan a fancy, formal dress-up party. When we first married, we said that if we lived to celebrate this day together, we would take a special trip. Then we would laughingly say, "somewhere that would accommodate our wheelchairs." After all, James would be eighty-one, and I would be seventy-three.

We're not doing either of these things today. This morning, James and I will be sitting in church with all of our children and grandchildren. The minister will recognize us from the pulpit today in honor of our anniversary. The children have ordered a floral arrangement in our honor for the altar table at the front of the church. Later, we will all go to lunch at a special restaurant the children have chosen.

The children offered to give us a beautiful reception at the church, but I felt it would be inappropriate because of James' advancing dementia. A party would be meaningless without his awareness of the significance of the occasion. Today will be a bittersweet day, I'm sure." (To be continued later).

10:00 P.M. "*This has been a wonderful day, this red-letter day in our marriage. We had a late lunch in a fabulous Japanese restaurant where the children had made reservations. Everyone had fun, especially our five grandsons. They were fascinated by the chef who prepared and served our meal. I enjoyed watching James have a good time. He is like a child in many ways. He was delighted by the "whole package" – the children, their joy, the atmosphere, the great food. He kept saying, "Whose birthday is it? Do we get cake?"*

The children have gone home. James, who was exhausted from all the activity and excitement, is in bed, sleeping soundly. Although, I, too, am tired, I am at my Bethel reflecting on the past fifty years. As I look at the picture of James that I keep here, I remember the way he was then, fifty years ago. He was so very handsome, so smart, so strong. He and I were inseparable, "joined at the hip." Although we had many friends and enjoyed doing things with them, we were content with one another. We have always been best friends. We have laughed together and cried together. We have worshiped together and prayed together. James has treated me like a Queen. I have never doubted that he loves me.

Today, on a day that should have been filled with shared memories of our life together, I am lonely for my sweetheart and best friend. I miss our sweet, intimate relationship, our companionship. I know that this day will pass and that God will give me the strength to go on. But just for today, I will grieve." *(Lucy)*

My Journal — December 31, 2007

"The year 2007 has been a year of subtle but steady decline in James' level of function. He can still do some things for himself, which I encourage. I want him to be as independent as is possible. I think this is crucial in helping him to maintain his dignity and self-esteem. It breaks my heart when he sometimes says, "I'm a nothing and a nobody."

I tease him and say, "You are the handsomest, most wonderful, brilliant and talented man in the world. You just want to hear me say that, don't you?" Then he grins. Thank You, Father, for that.

When I lay his clothes out, he can dress himself although he usually buttons his shirt wrong. As I come to the rescue and put the right buttons in the right buttonholes, I make a joke about it. I say, "Honey, you're just trying to start a new fad." He thinks that's funny.

Sometimes when I'm helping him dress, I think back to the day, fifty-one years ago when I fell in love with his reflection in a mirror. He was my "blind date" that day. He was the handsomest man I'd ever seen. His clothes were tailor-made, and they fit his trim body to perfection. That's why my heart broke the day I found my once perfectly groomed husband trying to put his legs into the sleeves of his shirt.

He said, "I don't know what's wrong. These pants must be too small." I tried to not let him see my tears as I removed the shirt and replaced it with his slacks. The saddest thing is to know that James will never be better in this world. He will only get worse, losing more and more of himself. I try to be positive as I help him live as normal a life as possible. This isn't easy when your heart is broken.

I know that there are those who love me and who, if they could, would gladly help me put back together the broken pieces of my heart, but they can't. Only God, the Mender -of- Broken Hearts, can do this. And He will.

In the new year, 2008, I plan to keep very close company with God the Father, trusting Him to watch over James and me, no matter what this new year holds for us." (Lucy)

As James and I began the year 2008, we were officially "homebound." Elsewhere in the book I talk about the reason for this. It's in the chapter on "Wisdom." Along with the responsibilities of caring for James, it seems that I am consistently facing one agonizing decision after the other. Much of the time, I feel totally inadequate and helpless.

Many times, I want to shout in frustration, "I can't do this anymore. I'm not strong enough or smart enough. I'm tired of facing all these decisions by myself." Sound familiar? Following is an excerpt from a journal entry that addresses that very issue.

My Journal — November 15, 2008

"I love the old hymns of my childhood and youth. Sometimes, during my long, sleepless nights, the words of one of them will come to me. Last night, it was the beautiful but haunting words: "Jesus walked this lonesome valley. He had to walk it by Himself. Nobody else could walk it for Him. He had to walk it by Himself."

Father, I know why You wanted me to remember those words last night. You wanted to remind me that Jesus willingly walked His valley so that I would never have to walk mine alone. You are telling me today that when I abide in You, You will abide in me. Thank You, Father, for this reminder.

I know the day is coming that I must face the inevitable. The time will come when I must make some difficult decisions concerning James' care, unthinkable choices that will require some "valley time." Whatever path God chooses, I know I will not be walking alone. Jesus, who understands better than anyone what it means to face the "unthinkable", will be walking with me. With His strength and courage as my example, I will say, "Not as I will, but as You will, Father." That's my prayer today. (Lucy)

My Journal — November 9, 2009

"Today is our fifty-second wedding anniversary. For some reason, all the sorrow, the loss, and the overwhelming challenges of the past ten years crashed over me like a tsunami, knocking me off my feet and threatening to wash me out to sea.

Ten years of bottled up tears began to flow this morning. They spilled out, running down my face, dripping off my chin, creating a mess. Through a decade of living with Alzheimer's disease, I have had to let go of so many dreams. The essence of James, the steady, loving, dependable force in my life is being erased – story-by-story, memory-by-memory. Everything that was familiar to him has faded into the unknown of this terrible disease. Thankfully, he always remembers me and the children.

Today, with no one here to share my grief and to comfort me, in desperation I dropped to my knees. Then I experienced a "supernatural awareness" of God's presence. I was covered, like a warm blanket, with His love and comfort. It was as if sorrow's icy grip on my heart melted away, and I was being held in my Heavenly Father's strong arms. In my heart, I heard Him saying, "Lucy, let go of the past. Keep all the good memories of the wonderful years you and James have shared. Now find new dreams on which to focus. I still have many good plans for your future. Trust Me and keep following me."

Although I didn't hear an audible voice, I know that today I have been on Holy Ground. With such a strong, loving Father leading me and helping me, I will continue to love and care for James as long as he needs me." (Lucy)

Perhaps this "supernatural encounter" with God the Father today has been orchestrated by Him so that I can comfort you with the comfort I have received. I pray that you will be encouraged and comforted as you experience your loneliness and heartache. Don't forget – you are never alone.

P.S. Although we can never recapture what is gone, we can embrace with love what remains.

I've already established that suffering and sorrow are a part of life. Knowing this, however, doesn't make it any easier to cope when we find ourselves in deepest, darkest trials. When all we have left is Jesus, we still have everything we need.

My Journal — October 5, 2011

"Father, today I'm "treading water in a river of tears," not really concerned or even caring that there may be rapids or waterfalls ahead. I don't feel guilty about my emotional meltdown and self-indulgence. I know in my heart that this "river" is being held in the palms of your strong hands. I am aware that at any moment, at any sign of danger, you will reach down, pick me up, gently dry me off and set me on a Solid Rock, Jesus Christ. I love that about You, Father. But for today, I must grieve – I know You understand this. Later, I will go to Clare Bridge and spend time with James. I know that our conversation, as we walk together in the garden there, will consist of the same questions and the same answers, but we will be together.

Last week, on October 1, when I was confronted with the reality of our choice, Yours and mine, to place James full-time in the care of others at Clare Bridge, I knew I would experience a new level of grief. On my way to take him there, I wanted to pick him up, hold him close to me and run away with him to escape the inevitable pain. I knew that wasn't the plan, but for a moment, I didn't care. When I go to see him now, so happy, surrounded by so many who genuinely love him and take such good care of him, I know we made the right choice. Thank You, Father, for sharing this burden of grief with me." (Lucy)

My Journal — February 2, 2012

"I read somewhere that grief sucks one's breath away, leaving one wondering if he or she will ever feel joy again. After I had placed James, my husband of fifty-four years, into a full-time care facility for Alzheimer's patients on October 1, 2011, I felt empty. I felt guilty, feeling that somehow I had failed him. Before he developed Alzheimer's, for forty-two years this man had been my strength, my protector, my encourager, my hero, my lover.

We loved being together. If for some reason we were apart for a few days, we could scarcely wait to be together again. Now I felt incomplete, as if I had lost my identity, my purpose for existing. Our house that I returned to that first night felt empty without him. So did my life. The only way I can describe that feeling is that I felt like I was in a "desert place, a barren nothingness." It was a new Season I now refer to as "a wasteland of emptiness." It described my empty house, my empty world, my empty bed. Except for a few exceptions, for the first time in fifty-four years, James was not with me at bedtime. I put off going to bed as long as I could, dreading the empty place next to mine. It seemed strange not to be responsible for getting anyone ready for bed except myself.

As difficult and exhausting as the past twelve years have been, I loved the fact that James was with me, especially at night. He always reminded me that he loved me, that he thought I was beautiful. He was funny and dear and precious, and I loved caring for him. Before going to sleep, he always said, "till death do us part. You remember that promise don't you?" He remembered that wedding day commitment even when he couldn't remember who or where he was.

That first night alone, before I went to sleep, I asked God to please keep him safe, to comfort him if he felt uneasy or frightened, to be sure he was warm, to put an angel in his room (and in mine.) After a night filled with strange, troubled dreams, I was up early. I spent a few minutes in prayer with my Heavenly Father. Then I quickly dressed and drove the short distance to where part of my "heart" now lives.

I was relieved to learn that James had slept well, not seeming anxious or depressed. They were having a little trouble getting him up for breakfast, however. I felt a little guilty hearing this because I had been letting him sleep as long as he wished. When I went into his room, he saw me and got so excited. He said, "There's my wife." I was happy to see that his favorite care associate (and mine) was assigned to care for him that day.

Together, we finally got him to the Dining Room, where he ate a huge breakfast of scrambled eggs, bacon, toast and jelly, cereal, milk and orange juice. James worried because I wasn't eating. Otherwise, he seemed content. He loved all the attention he was getting. That was one of the reasons I made the indescribably difficult decision to move him to Clare Bridge full-time. Thank You, Lord, for Your guidance."
(Lucy)

After that first day, I established a routine. I visited James at least twice a day, usually at his meal times so that I would not interfere with their excellent program: "Daily Moments of Success." Each morning there was a Bible Study, followed by exercise (Balloon toss, dancing); mental activities such as math and sentence completion: reminiscing; crafts.

I was greatly comforted by the loving care James was receiving, and the mental stimulation provided. It was something I had witnessed when he was spending the day there the fourteen months we lived in the building next door. Still, every time I left there I grieved. Sometimes I sat in my car and cried. Then I would remind myself, "I am doing this for James."

One day in late November 2011, in my nail salon, I picked up an old People magazine, dated February 28, 2011. On page forty-nine was a review, by Kim Hubbard, of Joyce Carol Oates' book, *A Widow's Story*. As I read it, I could scarcely believe how Oates' emotions following the death of her husband of forty-seven years paralleled mine. She said that for months, eating, sleeping, just getting through the "vast hideous Sahara of trackless time" that was each day, seemed impossible. She said that writing in her journals helped, writing that later became her book. (My goal.) Oates and her husband called each other "Honey" instead of by their names—something James and I have always done. They, too, rarely spent a night apart. Like James and me, they were inseparable. One priceless quote from the book will stay with me forever: "If we are asked, 'How are you?' we must not say, 'suicidal.' And you?"

Death is typically a clear starting point for grief, and it's clear that eventually there will be an end. But with dementia, loss and grief come in bits and pieces and can drag on and on for many years before the loved one dies. It is understandable why people often feel almost relieved after so many years of grieving. That is how I unashamedly felt when James died.

My Journal — February 11, 2012

My level of grief in these months following October 1, 2011, has perhaps lessened some, but grief is always here, just beneath the surface. At bedtime each night, as I look at my favorite picture of James taken a month after our wedding, (the one where he looks like a movie star), I'm surprised at the intensity of my pain. That small picture sitting on my bedside table is a reminder of the love we have shared for fifty-five years.

The grief I feel now is grief that began almost thirteen years ago when we heard the words, 'It's Alzheimer's'. Grief which has never ended. Grief that is always just there, impossible to escape, unavoidable. Sometimes the grief is profound. At other times, it's just a deep ache, a terrible loneliness. The Bible says that there is "a time to weep" (Ecclesiastes 3:4). But the Psalmist promises that even though we weep, "joy comes in the morning" (Psalm 30:5). That is so comforting to me during these long nights when it seems morning will never come. Thank You, Lord, for this provision." (Lucy)

I read somewhere, "When grief grabs our attention like a severe weather warning, our first thought may be, not only is a storm coming, but I'm not in control."

I believe that this is an excellent description of how grief works. Even now, a year after James' death, grief at times suddenly grabs my attention. As I'm working on this chapter, I tried to read some of it to my son. I found I couldn't do it without crying. I'm so grateful for the comfort God gives me for just such a time.

> You've kept track of my every toss and turn
>
> through the sleepless nights,
>
> Each tear entered in your ledger,
>
> each ache written in your book.
>
> Psalm 56:8 (*The Message*)

~ Courage ~

Today I'm searching for just the right words to share the truths I've learned the past thirteen years about God's provision of "courage." My first journal entries from July of 1999 documented our introduction to the real meaning of courage.

As James and I began this journey with Alzheimer's, we realized that it would require much faith and courage. We soon discovered that courage takes many forms, but it has only one origin: a deep, unshakable faith that God is continually and intimately present in our everyday personal lives. Think about it. He never lets us out of His Sight. He walks every step with us. God has proven that to me over and over in the past thirteen years.

Real courage, I've learned, originates deep within us from what is hidden in our hearts, placed there by God Himself. The history of our world is made up of stories of people who lived quietly, day after day, in the face of suffering, testing, and seemingly insurmountable problems. Most of us know or have known people whose lives have modeled this kind of courage for us. They are those who possess the kind of courage that perseveres when life crumbles and everything seems lost. When others would have given up in despair, they found their courage in their faith in God and His relentless love for them.

My personal role model of courage was my maternal grandmother, my Mamaw. When I hear the word "courage", my mind goes immediately to her, my "personal hero." In 1914, at the age of thirty-eight, my Mamaw was widowed when Pneumonia took the life of her strong, handsome husband. He was the love of her life. He adored her. He called her "Pet." I know this because I have some of the beautiful letters he wrote to her during their courtship. With five children depending on her strength, faith, and courage, she buried her sweetheart and put her trust in God. She drew the courage and strength she needed from her deep well of faith in Him.

For the next fifty-seven years, this beautiful, intelligent, cultured woman walked with the Lord, acknowledging His constant presence with her. She raised her children. She nurtured, adored, and helped raise her grandchildren. She farmed her land with the help of sharecroppers she hired and supervised. She learned to manage her finances, tithed her income, and opened her home to anyone who needed a refuge. She lived her life with "gusto", and her courage, faith, peace, and joy were contagious. As she opened her heart and home to her friends and loved ones, she taught me, by example, the importance of hospitality, friendship, and the joy of living. She lived consumed with her faith in God, her love for Him evident to everyone she met.

Mamaw's humble home was the favorite gathering place for her friends and family. Some of my sweetest childhood memories are of Christmases spent with her. As we traveled from our home to her farm in the country, we were looking forward to the love, the warmth, and the aroma of the wonderful food we would find there. Everyone loved going to her home. She gave great parties that included delicious food, singing around the piano and endless Domino games.

Mamaw did all of this while daily milking her numerous cows, (which she named), raising pigs and chickens for food, walking her fence line, planting and hoeing her large garden from which she gathered and canned fruits and vegetables for the winter. She also grew the prettiest flowers in the county. All this with only a cistern (a well) for water, which she drew, bucket by bucket, for all her needs.

Even as a child, God was teaching me courage and preparing me for the time in my life when I would need the kind of courage I saw in my Mamaw. From the age of eight to thirteen, I spent part of every summer with her. The memories of those summers I wouldn't trade for anything. Every Sunday morning we walked two miles through the woods (it was shorter than taking the road) to the little church she attended. I never heard her complain about the hot weather or the distance. She could always out walk me and outwork me. She had endless energy and strength and "miraculous" health. This is a blessing I am discovering in my senior years—a beautiful gift from God (and Mamaw).

During those memorable summers, I took baths in one of the big washtubs she filled every week on washday with water she drew from that cistern by her back porch. At night, I slept with her on her big feather bed, with the windows open to the sound of whip-poor-wills calling and wolves howling. I always felt safe with her. We prayed every night and each morning we read from her big Bible. She talked about God as if He were her best friend, which He was.

I'm thinking now, as I approach eighty years of age, alone for the first time in fifty-five years, of Mamaw's life. She was alone without her sweetheart from age thirty-eight to age ninety-five. I think about the loneliness, the fifty-seven years of nights, most of them spent alone as she aged. Her nearest neighbors were more than a mile away from her house. Her nights were spent without good locks on her door, with no Home Security System—only a bell in her yard to ring for help. Her security system was her faith in God, and that faith was the foundation of her courage. She taught me, as a child, that because of our faith in Jesus, we have a "guarantee", a promise from God found in Romans 8:1: "Therefore, there is now no condemnation for those who are in Christ Jesus."

Mamaw and I read *Romans, chapter eight,* often on those summer mornings spent with her. I still love that chapter. The promises contained there gave me great courage during the last weeks of James' life, our "Hospice Season." I referred to them during his funeral service, specifically Romans 8:38. "For I am convinced that neither death nor life, neither angels nor demons, neither the present nor the future, nor any powers, neither height nor depth, nor anything else in all creation, will be able to separate us from the love of God that is in Christ Jesus, our Lord."

One of Mamaw's favorite verses was Romans 8:37, which tells us "we are more than conquerors through Him who loved us." That promise means that victory is certain because of His great love for us. Mamaw would say, "Lucy Sue, because God loves you, failure is not possible when you trust in Him." Later, as a college student, when I had questions about my faith, these memories encouraged me to open my heart to Jesus and to receive His absolute, never-to-be-questioned—again assurance of my salvation.

When, at age ninety-five, Mamaw fell, breaking her hip, her faith sustained her until her neighbor found her the next day. That same faith was evident as she peacefully and gently died later from complications from her fall.

My grandmother's example of courage has sustained me and has certainly been a part of the foundation of my courage during my long, thirteen-year journey into the unknowns of Alzheimer's disease. I've said more than once during these years, "If Mamaw could do what she did, with God's help, I, too, can be strong and courageous."

"Mamaw, thank you for your legacy of courage and faith. I pray that I can leave the same legacy to my children and grandchildren. Your example has been a source of strength and courage for me all of my life, especially now. I'm learning as I travel my lonely road, that God uses circumstances, no matter how bleak or seemingly hopeless, to draw us closer to Him. Your life was a perfect example of this truth. I can scarcely wait to see you again, which I will."

Thank you for allowing me to share with you something so very special and personal to me. As I wrote about my grandmother's life, I realized again how powerful and loving our heavenly Father is; how He provides everything we need, just when we need it. There are so many lessons we can learn from one another, lessons we must pass on to those who follow behind us.

I pray that you, too, dear readers, have a "role model" of courage in your life story. Of course, we all have the perfect role model of courage in Jesus, the foundation of our courage.

Think with me for a moment about Jesus who was all God, but who chose to be clothed in flesh like ours that experienced hunger and thirst, weariness, loneliness, disappointment, rejection, fear, grief, and pain. When He was facing the cross, he experienced depression, dread, fear, and sorrow that almost killed Him when He thought about all that the Cross represented. Three times, in desperation, He begged His Father to "take away His cup of suffering." But with great courage and with the surrender of His will to the will of His Father, he prayed, "Not as I will, but as You will." He then rose from His knees and bravely faced, not just horrible physical suffering, but the terrible weight of all the sins of the world on His sinless body. Worst of all, He faced all this without His Father, who had to turn His back to Him at the time He needed Him most. That is something that we will never have to face. In light of what Jesus our Lord experienced, my problems seem small in comparison. His courage and His love flood my heart with courage.

"People seldom improve when they have
no other model but themselves to copy."
~Oliver Goldsmith.

My Journal — July 21, 1999

"*Tomorrow James has an appointment with a different neurologist, one who is on our new Medical Insurance. I have to admit —I'm a little anxious. We know that James has had a left frontal lobe stroke sometime in the past. This, however, does not explain the steady increase in his symptoms:*

- *His head never feels "right." In James' words, "It feels heavy and tight."*

- *Most mornings he is very "dizzy."*

- *His vision, "not the same." He had "floaters" in his right eye for two days.*

- *He experiences frequent anxiety and restlessness. His depression persists although he has been on the antidepressant, Zoloft, 100 mg daily, since February 4, 1999. His Cardiologist prescribed this.*

His memory is becoming more impaired. He has difficulty remembering:

- *how to use his bank card.*
- *how to balance his check book.*
- *location of items in our grocery store.*
- *which medication he takes, and when he takes it.*

I know that the fear I'm feeling is fear of the unknown. Not knowing what lies ahead is causing my imagination to magnify the possibilities until they are becoming "Giants."

God tells me over and over again in His Word, "Do not be afraid." "Be strong and courageous." "Do not fear." He promises to be with us, not matter what we're facing.

When Jesus was here on earth, he always reminded His followers, "Fear not." He knew that with faith in Him, his disciples could act with courage and confidence, even in the presence of fear and danger.

I know that it is only my absolute faith in God that will enable me to choose courage instead of fear. Today, I'm taking these steps to reinforce my courage for tomorrow and whatever the future holds:

- *I will meditate on God's promises in His Word—Most of them are already underlined and highlighted in my Bible.*

- *I will remember God's faithfulness to us in the past. We have been tremendously blessed and favored by God the Father.*

- *I will think about the courage of those "heroes" of faith in my life—My mother, my Mamaw, my sister.*

Speaking of "heroes," one of the best examples of courage is sitting in his recliner in our den. James Dishongh is not only the most righteous man I've ever known, he is one of the most courageous. I lean on him; I draw courage from him. His strength and courage are what gave me the confidence forty-two years ago to invest my life and future with him. (Of course, the fact that he looked like a movie star didn't hurt.) James has the courage of his convictions. His honesty and integrity are impeccable. Whatever God has required of him, he has done. He is strong and courageous because his hope is in the Lord; he walks and talks with Him daily. He is the "Spiritual Giant" of our family. I will draw my courage for tomorrow from him and our faithful Father.

My bible is open to Joshua 1:9, "Be strong and courageous. Do not be terrified; do not be discouraged, for the Lord your God will be with you wherever you go." God is saying that to me now. Thank You, Father." (Lucy)

My Journal — July 29, 1999

"Last week, on July 22, the doctor said these words to James, "I'm so sorry, but with your recent history and the result of the tests we did today, I believe it's Alzheimer's." I wanted to cover my ears and run away from the inevitable. All I could think about was how James' older sisters had lived the last years of their lives lost in a fog of the dementia of Alzheimer's. During their ten-year illness, at times the prospect of a genetic disorder terrified me.

On that day last week, our world was turned upside down by the word "Alzheimer's." Life as we knew it—the endless adventures, dreams yet unfulfilled, trips not yet taken—was washed away like children's sandcastles on the beach when the tides come in. All this week, with our worst fears realized, I have prayed consistently and unapologetically, that God would take away this bitter cup we are facing. When in simple faith we named our fears, He released the icy grip of fear from our hearts. In His Word, He assured us that we are not facing this frightening future alone. Through the prophet Isaiah's words in Isaiah 41:10, God made us this promise, "Do not fear, for I am with you; do not be dismayed for I am Your God. I will strengthen you and help you. I will uphold you with My righteous right hand."

When God says, "I will," I believe Him. He knows that what James and I are facing is unlike anything we've encountered before. He knows better than anyone how hard life can be. Because He is intimately acquainted with us, I am convinced that He will walk with us through all of the heartaches and struggles that lie ahead on our journey.

James is being his usual sweet, strong self. He keeps saying "It's going to be okay. We're going to trust God like we always have." My prayer today is, "Father, You know that all of this is beyond our understanding. Please give us wisdom and courage. Show us what to do, and guide us on this frightening journey into the unknown." (Lucy)

❦

My Journal — January 4, 2009

I've discovered during this past decade that fear is terribly destructive. It can hold us prisoner, robbing us of freedom, joy, and peace. Fear of the unknown can keep us on edge, waiting for the "nameless dread":

> *the next crisis,*

> *the next "New Normal",*

> *the next stage of Alzheimer's disease.*

I think the saddest thing about fear is that it makes us lose sight of the purpose and blessing of our calling as caregiver to our loved one. It robs us of the capacity to enjoy each day that we've been given with our "special someone." It prevents us from seeing the glimpses of beauty around us in nature and in simple acts and expressions of love.

In this new year, I'm taking a fresh stand against fear as James and I continue to face our "Giant", our "Goliath"— Alzheimer's. Jesus has set the standard of courage for me, and I will rise to that standard. I will firmly place my feet on the Rock of my Salvation, Jesus Christ, and stand tall against fear. I will shout at my "Giant." I will loudly proclaim that

God is still on the throne where He has always been. I will tell this "Goliath" and the watching world that God my Father is always victorious. He is incapable of losing, and He can bring me victory over fear.

As I take my stand and daily live out my faith, I believe that God will look at my life through His eyes of grace and reward my courage with more courage during these long, lonely, homebound months.

God just brought to my mind as I'm writing, that James is struggling against his own fears, his own "Goliath." Daily he faces physical weakness, social isolation, memory loss, confusion, depression and fear of the darkness. My goal is to help him by loving him fervently and unconditionally; by reassuring him; by creating a calm, safe environment; by never leaving him alone.

One thing I've learned the past ten years as James' Caregiver is that I only need enough courage for the moment. Knowing that God loves James and me unconditionally and forever, gives me the courage to get up each morning and face whatever challenges the day may hold.

Daily, I'm learning that everyone has some "Giant" that they must face at some time in their life. Everyone's "Giant" looks different, but somehow the same. They are all much bigger than we are, and they must all be fought with courage and faith, weapons that God has already provided.

Also, I know I must continue to hold tightly to God, clinging to Him as I have done from the beginning. I must believe that He hasn't finished my story until it is time—His time, His way. Like a constant, prevailing assurance, God remains with me. Everything else may slip away. My circumstances most certainly will change as time passes. But God never changes. He is the same yesterday, today, and forever. God never leaves me, forgets me or forsakes me. He is my Mighty Fortress, "a bulwark never failing." How do I know all this? His Word tells me so. Thank You, Father." (Lucy)

My Journal — September 11, 2009

"Today is the eighth anniversary of the worst terrorist attack in the history of America. James and I are watching Fox News on television. As I listen to those helping us remember and relive that day, I am once again amazed at the stories of unbelievable strength and courage that are being shared. We are hearing story after story of real heroes, and I am reminded of the inner invincibility of the human spirit. I am encouraged by their courage and strength that continues today, eight years later, and which enables them to endure the unendurable.

One widow, standing at the microphone with her children, made this statement, "In times of trouble, we are forced to lean on the Lord, to become dependent but also stronger, more resilient." As she spoke, God spoke those words to my heart.

James keeps saying, "What's happened? Why are those people running?" I remind him that this happened in New York City eight years ago. I also remind him that we were in New York City and went to Ground Zero in 2002 on our Guided Tour. He doesn't remember any of this, but I will never forget. Neither will the fathers, mothers, sisters, brothers, wives, husbands, children of those who gave their lives that day. Many of them died so that others could live. I'm claiming this kind of courage for James and me today. Thank You, Father." (Lucy)

~ Directions and Instructions ~

Remember me, the "non-risk-taker"? Before I leave home, I want detailed instructions and directions, with very visible landmarks and an excellent map. I'm grateful that God Himself is handling the traveling plans for this journey into the unknown of Alzheimer's.

Even though we can't see the whole path, we have the greatest Guide we could ask for, the Lord God Almighty. He not only guides us by His Spirit, He has given us the most excellent Guide Book ever written, the Bible, His inspired Word. He has given us, through His word, a light for our path. The psalmist tells us, "By your words I can see where I'm going; they throw a beam of light on my dark path. I've committed myself, and I'll never turn back from living by Your righteous order" (Psalm 119:105 *The Message*.)

Earlier in that same Psalm, we find this assurance: "You're blessed when you stay on course, walking steadily on the road revealed by God. You're blessed when you follow His directions, doing your best to find Him. That's right - you don't go off on your own; you walk straight along the road he set" (Psalm 119: 1-3, *The Message*).

On every other trip James and I have taken, we always knew where we were going. We might decide, occasionally, to take the scenic route, but we always had a good road map. Therefore, we knew where we were and that we would eventually reach our original destination. On this journey with Alzheimer's, God has not handed us a detailed road map. He wants us to trust Him to do the guiding and directing. I have to remind myself constantly that when I trust God with our itinerary, I don't need a travel plan. He will, with His love and wisdom, take James and me to the place He has prepared for us.

God tells us that when we obey His laws and instructions for us, we are blessed. We can confidently stay on the path He has given us to walk when we trust and follow Him. Psalm 119:35 (*The Message*) says: "Guide me down the road of your commandments; I love traveling this freeway." I love this scripture.

As you know, I talk a lot about being a non-risk-taker, as if it's something to be proud of. It isn't. It's saying that I don't trust God to take care of me, and that isn't true. What is true is that I was sheltered much of my life. I was a quiet, gentle little girl, with parents who protected me as much as possible from the burdens and ugliness of life. We were poor during those Depression years, but I didn't know it. My mother could make the most of whatever she had to work with, and we were very blessed. Later, when I met and married James, he too sheltered me. He didn't want me to worry about anything, especially financial matters, which he handled brilliantly.

As I matured and encountered the typical difficulties that are part of living, I began to ask God to open my eyes to the things He wanted to do through me. I discovered that He had created in me so much more potential than I was exhibiting in my life. As I searched more deeply to find His will and direction for me, I found the courage I needed to become a risk-taker for Him.

Following my "Damascus Road" experience with Jesus in my college dorm in January of 1954, God immediately began to place in my heart the plans He had for me. With His direction and guidance, I left college at the end of the fall semester and enrolled in Lillie Jolly School of Nursing in Houston, Texas.

One day, in the midst of all these life changes, God reminded me that I was now a child of the King with all the privileges of a Princess. That meant that I could have an audience with my Father, the King, at any time. I could come into His presence with every need, every request, knowing that He would be loving and wise in all of His decisions for me. I could be confident that He would always provide just what I needed and even more than I would request. This realization of my position in the kingdom became my spiritual foundation that helped to prepare me for this arduous journey.

From the beginning of that new-found relationship with the Lord to the present, my life has not been without bumps and hurdles. However, even in the hard times, I've had the comfort of His promises and His presence.

Romans 5:3-4 tells us, "We continue to shout our praise even when we're hemmed in with troubles, because we know how troubles can develop passionate patience in us, and how that patience forges the tempered steel of virtue, keeping us alert for whatever God will do next" (*The Message*).

I've discovered that when I feel lost and life seems to be spinning out of control, it's because I've temporarily taken my eyes off the Lord, My Guide, my source of peace and direction. When this occurs, He picks me up, gently brushes me off, and sets me back on the path He has planned for me.

My Journal — September 25, 2009

It's very late, but while James is sleeping soundly, for the moment, I want to write down some thoughts. I'm sitting in my recliner in our bedroom, a floor lamp lighting my journal as I write.

As we continue this journey, I know that God is at work twenty-four hours a day. I never doubt that He directs our paths, even when we can't see the evidence. When our journey began, I had more questions than answers. I tried very hard to not ask "why?" although that is a typical human reaction to the things we don't understand. One day, the Holy Spirit pointed out a Scripture, Deuteronomy 29:29: "The secret things belong to the Lord our God." My amazed response was, "Of course they do."—and I praised Him.

It's wonderful knowing that I have a Big God who is in control, even when I don't understand. I especially need that assurance at this point in our journey. There are times lately when I feel alone and lost in this wilderness of James' advancing dementia.

Being lost is a terrible thing. We've all heard stories of individuals who were separated from their party and were lost in the wilderness. Many had happy endings, but others ended tragically, with the lost one never found or found too late. Stories of lost children are the most tragic. For this reason, I was very protective of our small sons.

One day, I took my youngest son to a store in a local mall where I regularly shop. While I shopped, I was careful to keep him close to me. That particular day, however, I suddenly realized he was no longer playing hide-and-seek with me from under the clothes rack. Terrified, I started running, asking all the sales people and other shoppers to help me look for him.

After a few desperate moments, one of the salesmen called out, "I've found him." Weak with relief, I finally saw him. He was standing by the UP escalator. With his hands on his hips, he said, "I was just trying to decide if I should ride up." I couldn't stop hugging him.

Even now, when I think of that day forty years ago, my chest gets tight with the "What if?" of that day. I felt the same way in December of 2008 when I lost James in the small mall near our home.

I felt that way today, coming home with James after a busy morning of running errands. We were both tired and hungry. Also, I was stressed by James' confusion and endless questions and by the strange sounds coming from our aging car. As we stopped at a traffic light near home, I suddenly felt "lost", alone in the world, unprotected, fragile, and vulnerable. At that moment, I felt overwhelmed and weighed down under the burden of the responsibilities of caring for James, our car, our house, our finances. It was as if everything came crashing down around me. I was "off the trail," hopelessly "lost in the wilderness" of our circumstances. I wanted someone to find me, to hold me, to reassure me, to tell me what to do. I desperately needed help to find the "on ramp" back to the road to hope. Thankfully, I knew where to find the help I needed.

With all these emotions almost smothering me, we arrived home where I fed James, took him to the bathroom and settled him in his recliner for a nap. He was asleep almost immediately.

Without stopping to eat, I hurried to my blue chair, my "Bethel where I always feel safe and comforted. There, I poured out my feelings to the Lord—all the fears, the insecurity, the helplessness, the lostness. As I prayed, I could imagine Jesus standing there with His arms opened wide. I picked up my Bible and opened it to a scripture passage I could have recited from memory Matthew 11:28-30: "Come to me, all you who are weary and burdened, and I will give you rest. Take my yoke upon you and learn from me, for I am gentle and humble in heart, and you will find rest for your souls. For my yoke is easy, and my burden is light."

God is so amazing. In my Bible, beside this verse, I had written Psalm 55:22. The Psalm that I read and studied earlier this week was Psalm 55. I had highlighted verse 22: "Cast your cares on the Lord and He will sustain you; he will never let the righteous fall."

I knew this was no coincidence. God was sending me clear instructions through His word—not once, but twice. He was very careful to see that I received them. "Thank You, Father, for your incredible love."

This has been a very long, exhausting day. I finally ate lunch, although I had been spiritually fed by my Heavenly Father as I spent time with Him at my Bethel. That time spent with Him had given me the attitude adjustment I so desperately needed.

This evening, with fresh hope and strength, I was able to lovingly and patiently care for my precious James. We ate hot dogs, ice cream, and chocolate chip cookies for dinner—not too healthy but so much fun.

Then we snuggled on the couch and watched the Fox News Channel, James' favorite. He enjoys the evening lineup: Bill,

Sean, and Greta. He thinks of them as friends. He especially likes Greta, but he is too sleepy tonight to watch her show. I helped him brush his teeth and get ready for bed. He's there now, breathing softly, looking so dear, so child-like, as he sleeps. As I watch him, my heart "hurts" with my love for him. I'm so grateful that God has "called me" to care for this wonderful, godly man.

Now, I too, will finally go to bed, confident that Jesus Himself and the angels are watching over us through the night. Someone has said, "We are never so lost that angels can't find us." I love that." (Lucy)

Are you facing a situation where you want to trust God, but you feel lost? Does the path ahead seem dark and dangerous and unfamiliar? Hopefully, it has helped to read about my feelings and emotions which I have shared with you as honestly as I know how. I want you to discover, as I have, that you are not alone in the things you're feeling and experiencing. I pray that what God is teaching me during these indescribably difficult days of caregiving will encourage you during yours.

My Journal — February 1, 2010

I'm at my Bethel very early this morning. I tossed and turned all night, my mind bombarded by troubling thoughts. I know that change is coming; that it is inevitable. The time is approaching rapidly to take the next step in James' care. As painful as it is to admit, I know I can no longer keep doing this on my own. When the time does come, God will walk us through the decisions to be made. I have no doubts about this. I know that the process of waiting for His answers will be difficult, and the answers, heartbreaking. The next step whatever it is, is going to require a radical, risk-taking kind of faith to get through the "I don't understand, but I will trust You, Lord" moments.

As I'm writing, I'm thinking of others who have waited for God's answers and instructions for their next step and how God answered their questions: All the "heroes of faith" named in the book of Hebrews, all the Old Testament Prophets (major and minor), the Psalmist, Mary and Joseph, the disciples, the Apostle Paul.

For some reason, I'm thinking about Habakkuk, one of the minor prophets. I always loved the fact that he faithfully stood in his "watch tower" waiting for God's answer to his difficult questions. As I turn now to the short, three-chapter book of Habakkuk, I see the words I wrote in the margins of the first chapter on July 22, 2002: "It is always wise to wait for God's answer." I wrote these words exactly three years after we received James' diagnosis, "Alzheimer's."

In Habakkuk 2:3 (The Message), God says, "If it is slow in coming, wait. It's on its way. It will come right on time." I'm learning every day on this strange journey that God is always at work. He shows up in my daily circumstances with His answers—never too late, but right on time.

My prayer today: "Father, You know that I am facing a critical time in our journey. I don't have any answers, but I know You do. You chose a burning bush in a desert wilderness to give Moses Your directions and instructions for his future. Sometimes I wish I could have a "burning bush" in which I could clearly hear your directions for our future. But I know that You have chosen to speak to me through Your inspired Word, the Bible. It's a book You wrote for me, and I love reading it. There in its pages, I "hear" Your words cutting through my confusion and my "this doesn't make sense" moments. In faith, I will search for Your answers to all my questions. I will wait for Your loving directions and instructions for James and me.

Although I'm a little nervous, knowing that Your answer may not be what I would have chosen for myself, I will trust You. Since beginning this journey, I've spent enough time in Your Presence, Father, to know that You are trustworthy and faithful. I look back and see that each step has been a progression to the next part, which we're traveling one step at a time. It's enough to know that You're walking each step with us. Even though our future is unknown, You are not. You are a familiar Friend, and this truth so humbles me. Today, I am thanking You with a full heart." (Lucy)

As we face the unknown ahead on our journey, there is one thing we can know: God has already provided for our future. The Apostle Paul, in Philippians 4:19, tells us: "And my God will meet all your needs according to His glorious riches in Christ Jesus." When God the Father says that He will do something, we can know that He will.

Wherever you are on your journey, you can trust that God knows where you are and where your next step will lead you. Although you, too, may have reached your "this doesn't make sense" moment, wait for God's instructions. When you do, you'll never need to regret your decisions.

Sometimes the greatest obstacle to following God is our longing to know what the outcome will be. The truest test of faith is going forward without knowing. The Good Shepherd's plan is to take care of us, to meet our needs, to protect us. I've read that a good shepherd will relentlessly search for a lost lamb. When that lamb continually goes off on its own, the shepherd may choose to break one of its legs. Then the shepherd places the lamb on his shoulder and tenderly carries it until it learns total dependence on him. In the same way, when we fail to follow the Lord in obedience and we go off on our own, He will find us, pick us up and carry us close to His heart until we learn to trust Him. The Lord knows that unless we trust Him, we won't follow Him. Trusting God is the key to reaching the destination He has chosen for each of us.

My Journal — March 2, 2010

"Today at my Bethel, the reality and the specter of change is filling my thoughts. Life is all about change. It always has been. It always will be. No matter how carefully and thoughtfully we plan our course, changes are inevitable. I'm a person who prefers order and a well-written script with an intriguing, uplifting plot that ends with the words, "They lived happily ever after." Instead, the words, "it's Alzheimer's" rudely interrupted our orderly world, abruptly changing our carefully planned script.

Ten years ago life as James and I knew it was changed forever. The threads that had so carefully woven the tapestry of our lives began to unravel. Sadly, I couldn't seem to find a way to stop the frightening process. I had always trusted God, even as a child, to fix whatever was broken in my life. Now my faith and trust were being tested as never before.

Had God the Father actually orchestrated the changes that were disrupting our safe, predictable world? Was He fully aware of our situation? My mind wanted to ask these questions, but my heart already knew the answer: He is the same faithful Father He has always been. He is still the Mender-of-broken things. He is still the One who said in Malachi 3:6, "I, the Lord do not change." In absolute faith, I reached out to my Father.

Today, I'm preparing to do the "unthinkable", to sell my miracle-from-God house. For weeks, I have been standing at a crossroad on our journey, waiting for directions from our Guide. For the past six months, I've been trying to convince myself that I'm okay, that I can endure. During these months my Gracious Father has provided the supernatural health, strength and energy that I have needed to care for James, our home, our car, our finances, the shopping. He has given me wisdom for all the decision making. However, I could sense that God has been leading me to take this next step, even though it is a monumental test of my common sense.

I know that our children and our friends have been very concerned about my physical and emotional well-being. The time has come when I'm not sleeping more than four or five hours each night. Sometimes I forget to eat, resulting in a steady weight loss. This physical toll, along with the emotional stress and loneliness of being homebound, has finally brought me to this crossroad, this fork in the road.

Every January 1 prayerfully select a "word" for the year. My word for the year 2010 is "surrender." I know now why the Holy Spirit led me to choose this word. Romans 8:14 tells us that the true children of God are those who let God's Spirit lead them. And, that is exactly what I'm going to do. After all, I am a 'true child' of God." (Lucy)

Little did I know when I wrote this journal entry that God had already prepared the way and worked out all the details for our move. God the Father, the Miracle Worker and our Guide, had drawn the blueprints and had covered every step with His providential care. My part of the process was to trust Him and to surrender to His instructions and directions.

I must confess that once the decision was made to take this enormous step, there were many anxious moments. At times, I questioned my sanity. According to the plan, I would be selling our "miracle-house", our Rainbow Bend "dream house" filled with the things I had so carefully and lovingly collected during the past fifty-three years. James and I would be moving into a two-room apartment in a Brookdale Assisted Living Community, The Hampton at Pearland. This community contains three lovely two-story homes and a highly acclaimed Memory Care facility, Clare Bridge, where James would spend a part of each day.

I knew that this was God's plan, the one I had prayed for during many hours spent on my knees in prayer. As painful as all these changes were, I knew they were the answer to our needs. I had come to the place where taking James anywhere often ended in disaster and always in exhaustion and frustration for both of us. I am so grateful for a Heavenly Father, who knows what is best for us. I know that His relentless love will give me the wisdom and courage to follow the path He has laid out for me. I will keep His "guide-book", the Bible, nearby and refer to it daily so that I won't stray from the path He has chosen. By following His directions for me, I am assured of reaching my destination—the one He has already prepared for me.

My prayer for you is that you, too, will have the wisdom to surrender to God's plan for you and the faith to follow that plan, wherever it leads. Remember, we have a Mighty God, and nothing is too hard for Him.

~ Endurance and Patience ~

The words "endurance" and "patience" make me a little nervous. They seem to suggest that I may be facing a tough time in the future. They make me think that there may also be some work involved.

Our Father knew when He packed these provisions for our journey with Alzheimer's that they were virtues we would desperately need at some point along the way. When we face trials, He knows that our first response, the typical response, is to run as far away as possible. But we read in His Word that He has a different plan. He says to us, "Wait for me."

"Waiting" is another word that has negative "vibes" for me. I don't like to wait. Does anyone? I'm always in a hurry, with more "things" to do than I have hours to do them. Whether we like it or not, much of life here on earth is spent waiting:

We wait for traffic lights to change.

We wait for the thunderstorm to pass (as I'm doing now).

We wait for the doctor to see us—finally.

We wait for the check in the mail.

We wait for results of diagnostic tests.

One of the hardest waits I ever endured was waiting for the results of Psychological testing that would ultimately tell us that James had Alzheimer's. We were both devastated by this diagnosis, knowing a little of what it entailed. For the past twelve years, we had seen first-hand and up-close what Alzheimer's had done to the lives of James' two older sisters and their loved ones. It broke James' heart to watch his beautiful, intelligent, big sisters gradually, over the course of about ten years, become almost unrecognizable in their dementia. Once, when we were visiting the younger of the two, about a year before her death, her confusion was very apparent. The once beautifully groomed, poised and confident former bank vice-president was now aimlessly wandering around, looking for her keys, looking for her daughter, asking endless questions. Seeing the loss of who she once had been broke our hearts. James turned to our son and said, "If this ever happens to me, shoot me." When first one and then the other died, it saddened us, but we were so grateful that they were with God in Heaven, healed and whole once more.

As the months passed, after James' diagnosis, I realized that living with Alzheimer's was like living in a vacuum, never knowing what the day would bring. I felt that I was always waiting, "waiting for the other shoe to drop," waiting for any signs of change in my sweet James. As a result I became almost paranoid, "anticipating" I wasn't sure "What"? I did know that changes would eventually come. Not being able to make plans for the future, in the light of this knowledge, was hard to accept. Unrealized, unfulfilled dreams became a sad reality. It was only through our faith in God and His promises that James and I were able to move forward, determined to live each day trusting in Him. When we began nurturing our waiting with our faith in God and His plan, our waiting was rewarded with more patience and endurance. Together we prayed and made a decision to turn this tragedy into an opportunity to honor God and to demonstrate His faithfulness to us. We wanted those who were watching to see our faith and endurance lived out through our response to this disruptive moment in our lives.

~ Exercising Endurance ~

God's Word tells us "love endures all things." (1 Corinthians 13) Does that mean all the unmentionable, unimaginable "drudgery" of caring for our loved one? Does it mean the long, sleepless, stress-filled nights when our loved one

asks a million questions,

roams around the room looking for 'something',

can't find the bathroom,

asks over and over again if he's safe, and

doesn't know 'who' or 'where' he is?

Does it mean the days your loved one gets up and eats five bananas while you have gone to take a shower? Could it mean the constant heartache and sadness, the constant exhaustion, the constant anxiety?

The answer to all the above is, "Yes." Whether we understand it or not, that is exactly what it means: "ALL things."

The circumstances we encounter as caregivers will always challenge our endurance. Many times we may feel a desperate need to run away, to escape our "prison." Other times we may be tempted to run ahead of God, trying to endure our trials in our own strength. At these times, we need to remember: "nothing is impossible with God" (Luke 1:37). God has promised us a "breakthrough", but He has a timetable for this. When we are "out of gas" and "running on fumes", we can confidently ask for help. Then the Holy Spirit will fill us with supernatural strength and endurance. This isn't a "hollow" promise. It is a fact.

Anytime I get discouraged, I think of Paul and Silas in a cold, hard prison cell in Philippi. "About midnight Paul and Silas were praying and singing hymns to God, and the prisoners were listening to them" (Acts 16:25). Paul's entire life following his Damascus road transformation was a model of endurance. Out of his suffering and trials came the beautiful "prison letters" that tell us everything we need to know about God's faithfulness in every situation. When I read these, especially his letter to the Philippians, I thank him for his faith, courage, and endurance. I say to myself, "If Paul could do what he did, demonstrating not only patience but contentment, I can do the same."

I want to conclude these thoughts about endurance with an incredible story from Carelinks, January, 2011. This is a monthly publication from *"Interfaith CarePartners,"* to Care Team members. The story is a graphic illustration of the endurance and resilience available to those who find themselves in a "hole," either as a full time caregiver or as a victim of Alzheimer's, as our loved one must feel at times. Here is the story:

The Farmer's Donkey: A Pastoral Fable

One day a farmer's donkey fell down into a well. The animal cried piteously for hours as the farmer tried to figure out a way to get him out. Finally he decided it was probably impossible, and the animal was old and the well was dry anyway, so it just wasn't worth it to try and retrieve the donkey. So the farmer asked his neighbors to come over and help him cover up the well. They all grabbed shovels and began to shovel dirt into the well.

At first, when the donkey realized what was happening he cried horribly. Then, to everyone's amazement, he quieted down and let out some happy brays. A few shovel loads later, the farmer looked down the well to see what was happening and was astonished at what he saw. With every shovel of dirt that hit his back, the donkey was shaking it off and taking a step up.

As the farmer's neighbors continued to shovel dirt on top of the animal, he continued to shake it off and take a step up. Pretty soon, to everyone's amazement, the donkey stepped up over the edge of the well and trotted off.

If we want to be triumphant in the face of our adversities, we can take lessons from the donkey and use them as stepping-stones to victory.

~ Practicing Patience ~

There is nothing that is more needed in the life of an Alzheimer's caregiver than the virtue of patience. Take it from me—an "authority" on the subject.

A caregiver's patience requires time, commitment, and practice, practice, practice. Practicing patience is not the same as resigning ourselves to the inevitable trials ahead. Patience is the ability God will give us to meet with calmness, endurance and peace the trials and testing we will encounter. It is the surrender of our disappointments and unfulfilled dreams to His greater plan for us. It believes that He always has a reason for every obstacle and delay He allows on our life's journey.

Most important of all, patience requires constant dependence on God, demonstrated by prayer and quiet times spent with Him in His Word. Since patience is a fruit of God's Spirit Who comes to live with us at the time of our salvation, we only need to claim it. God has a "bumper crop" of patience, and He will never grow impatient with us when we ask for it.

Patience is a gift of God's love. I'm so glad that His Word paints for me a picture of a loving Father who is patient with me, even at times when my attitudes and actions don't reflect inward peace and outward control.

My dear friend, Don Piper, in his book, "Heaven is Real", reminds us that God never promises that life will be easy. He quotes the Apostle Paul, who, in his letter to the Colossian Christians, tells them that with God's power, they can endure. Paul writes, "We also pray that you will be strengthened with all His glorious power so that you will have all the endurance and patience you need" (Colossians 1:11, NLT).[15]

Don and Paul are experts on the importance of practicing patience in any and every circumstance. With their example, I will run my race with patience, keeping my eyes on Jesus, the author and perfector of my faith.

Fellow caregiver, I know that sometimes we can't see beyond the demands of the moment, the lack of sleep, the exhaustion, the

15   Don Piper and Cecil Murphy, *Heaven is Real*, Penguin Group, Berkley Publishing Group, 375 Hudson, New York, NY, 2007.)

loneliness, and the stress. But always, during the long, dark nights when discouragement and sadness threaten to smother me, God reaches down in love to comfort and encourage me. He repeatedly assures me that everything I'm experiencing is important to Him. He knows that when James is up during the night, running into things, looking for something, I need extra patience. Although I have trouble wrapping my mind around such love, I am wonderfully strengthened by it and by the reality that God will supply all the patience I need to be a loving, gentle caregiver to James.

Will I always be patient? No. Does that mean that I'm a miserable failure? No. It simply means that I must take a deep breath, let it out slowly, and then rest in the Lord. I do this by spending time with Him in prayer and listening as He speaks to me through His Word. With His help, I can then start over. With all my heart, I want to be the patient caregiver He has called me to be. I can trust that with God's help patience will be a natural outflow of the desire that is already in my heart.

Through the years, I journaled my emotions as I dealt with the toll that Alzheimer's was taking on James and me. It helped to write down my feelings, read them, and then surrender them to God. I always tried to be brutally honest, knowing that God already knew everything I was feeling; everything I was facing and would face in the years ahead. Following are a few entries dredged from the mines of my anxiety, exhaustion, frustration, and heartache.

$$\text{\large ❧}$$

My Patience and Endurance Journal Entries From 2000-2011

My Journal — November 30, 2000

"Father, it seems that almost daily I am faced with a new problem. Today, I'm considering trading our two vehicles for

a new car. Sometimes, instead of stopping to talk to You about it, my mind says, "I can figure this out by myself." All the time, You are saying, "Be patient, Lucy; wait for me." When I stubbornly and impatiently run ahead of You, and do what my mind tells me rather than listening to You, I seem to be saying by my action, "I don't need You." I am so sorry, Father. This not only dishonors You, but the results of my decision have all the marks of a do-it-yourself project. I always need You, Father. Please forgive me and help me to wait patiently for You to give me Your answers to my problems." (Lucy)

My Journal — December 1, 2000

"Father, as I'm reading over yesterday's journal entry, I realize how ridiculous some of my worries and thoughts are in light of Your love for me. I know that I can do nothing in my strength. Today, I'm making a new commitment to wait for You, (patiently), and to accept Your timetable, not mine. My prayer today is, "Oh Father, I can't." I believe that these words are sweet to Your ears because You know they are spoken out of my surrendered heart. They mean that I depend entirely on You. I know this has been Your plan for me since the beginning of this journey. Thank You for lovingly waiting for me to discover it. And thank You for sending the perfect person to help us with the task of trading and buying a new car." (Lucy)

My Journal — Friday, October 4, 2002

James and I are so excited. Tomorrow morning at 6:30 we are leaving on a Guided Bus Tour up the East Coast to see the Fall foliage. It is a trip we had always planned to take but didn't want to take alone. Now we will be with much loved, longtime friends from a previous church. The Tour Guide is also a familiar friend, a former church staff member.

I've been packing for days, trying to be very organized and thoughtful. I've been making lists, something I love doing. Packing, for me, is half the fun of a trip. I decided to take two large suitcases, one for each of the two weeks. That way, we would only need to deal with one suitcase at a time.

I've made an extra special effort to be patient with James on these very busy last few days. Tuesday, I called to stop the newspaper for two weeks. Then I went to our Post Office to stop our mail for two weeks. Wednesday, I took James for a haircut, and today I'm getting a haircut. I'm taking James with me because he sometimes unpacks the suitcases when I'm not watching. Thankfully, I have everything of his (and mine) packed in individual large Ziploc plastic bags, one for each day of the trip. I'm quite impressed with my ingenuity. (Forgive my pride, Lord.)

I'm a little nervous about taking James so far away from his familiar setting (and from a convenient bathroom). I know that this trip is going to require a lot of patience on my part, and I've already talked to God the Father about this. As I've shared my concerns with our fellow travelers, they have assured me that they will help whenever I need them. The men have promised to help me with our luggage and with getting James to the restroom and back safely to the bus at each rest stop. This assurance has given me peace about my decision to take this much-needed vacation. At this church, James had been, for forty years, a strong, spiritual leader with a servant's heart. I know that these dear friends love us, and we treasure them. I can scarcely wait until we're on our way." (Lucy)

My Journal — Friday, October 21, 2002

"James and I returned home yesterday from our "awesome" trip. We were exhausted but filled with wonderful memories.

The men traveling with us were true to their promise; they took excellent care of James. He had only a couple of "incontinence accidents" which were unavoidable, and everyone was so patient and understanding. There was only one thing that "tried" my patience. Every night for fourteen nights, after James and I had gone to bed, we had to get up, sometimes several times and look at the clothes he would be wearing the next day. It was an ongoing obsession with him.

It would have been so easy to lose patience with him because I was always exhausted by bedtime, but I had prayed for an extra measure of endurance and patience and God faithfully granted it. Thank You, Father." (Lucy)

My Journal — January 20, 2003

"At my Bethel this morning I turned in my Bible to the "love chapter," 1 Corinthians 13. Verse four reads, "Love is patient, love is kind." I remember a minister suggesting that when reading verses four through seven, we should substitute our name in place of the word "love." There is a note in my Bible where I have written, "Lucy is patient, Lucy is kind." It was a wake-up call for me. I've noticed

that James is becoming very sensitive to my moods and even my expressions. I want always to show my love to him by my patience and tenderness.

Father, this morning I'm asking You to help me control my emotions and my responses to the unexpected "messes" and occurrences of each day. Today I fussed at James for breaking one of my favorite cups. I surrender to You my stress, my anxiety, and my occasional lack of patience. I know that without Your help, I will totally "blow it," something I never want to do. My lack of patience causes James to be stressed. He already feels insignificant, uneasy, and insecure. I never want him to feel guilty about his lack of judgment and his occasional incontinence, something over which he has no control. My goal at this point in our journey is to create a loving, stress-free, peaceful atmosphere for him. With Your help, Father, I know I can accomplish this. I love James so much, and I know You love him even more." (Lucy)

My Journal — February 8, 2005

"Last week, the mattress store delivered our new Tempur-Pedic beds. When we bought them, I was so excited. We bought twin-size mattresses and adjustable platforms. I decided on twin-size because:

They are easier to handle.

One can be adjusted without the other.

They can be used as singles.

They would take the place of a hospital bed if needed.

When the deliverymen brought them in, they were not sure that they would fit inside the frame of our beautiful king-size four-poster bed, but they did. Of course, they did. I had prayed that they would. I put twin-size fitted sheets on each mattress. Then I used our king-size sheets and bedspread. When bedtime came, we eagerly climbed into bed. I was anticipating comfort and freedom from back and hip pain. The bed felt wonderful. I was talking to James about what a wise decision we had made when he said, "This mattress is broken. It has a crack in the middle." I tried to explain to him that the "crack", which was barely noticeable, was the necessary space between two mattresses placed side-by-side. James got out of bed, saying, "I can't sleep in this broken bed." He was adamant about it, and he slept in his recliner the rest of the night. Thankfully, by the next night, I had convinced him that the bed was not broken. After that first night, when James had decided it was okay to sleep there, I would occasionally say, "Isn't our new bed wonderful?" And he would say, "I love it. It's so wonderful." Thank You, Father, for patience." (Lucy)

My Journal — January 27, 2007

"Yesterday morning James had laser surgery for Prostate Cancer. Because it was Day Surgery, we came home last night. James has an indwelling catheter that has become my new "challenge." It has been a twenty-four hour a day, minute-by-minute job to keep him from pulling out the catheter. He is insistent that he must remove it to go to the bathroom. He can't understand that the tube is there for that purpose. I ended up sleeping in a chair beside the bed to keep him from getting up and dismantling the whole apparatus,—the bag and catheter. He became very upset

with me because I "couldn't understand that he must get up and go to the bathroom." This morning, I am sitting in our bedroom in my recliner next to his recliner, watching him "like a hawk." Earlier this morning, I took him into the bathroom and let him watch as the urine went through the catheter into the commode. He was fascinated, but within minutes he had forgotten the "visual", and we are back where we started. I have a feeling that the next few days may be one of the greatest tests of patience in history.

Father, thank You for the knowledge that You will give me the strength and patience I need to endure the next few days calmly until this catheter is removed." (Lucy)

❧

My Journal — April 19, 2011

"Father, I am at my wits end. I can't do this alone. I know this. I know I must always lean on You, knowing that whatever I'm doing for James, I am doing for You. But sometimes I let my frustrations and impatience win. When this happens, I am less than loving and patient with James. Please forgive me. James' eczema on his arms is so bad, even with medication. He constantly scratches them and makes them bleed. I'm spending a lot of money on great first aid supplies, which I carefully and skillfully apply. Then James swiftly and skillfully removes them, the first time my back is turned. Sometimes, when we get into bed, I remind him not to touch his arms or the bandages. He cheerfully says "Okay." In a few minutes, I hear him moving around, and I'll say, "James are you touching the bandages?" He'll say, "No." But when I get up to check, the bandages are pushed down his arms forming "bracelets" on his wrists. Needless to say, my patience has had a good workout by then. Also, the sheets and his T-shirt are now white with red spots. I

laughingly told him recently that I would start buying red sheets and shirts and stop stressing. He said, "that's a great idea." Father, please heal James' eczema and help me to be more patient with the sweetest, most unselfish person I've ever known." (Lucy)

☙❧

My Journal — Monday, May 30, 2011

"James is very sick this morning. He coughed all night and, as a result, we were both awake all night. We are at the doctor's office now because he is "working us in." We could have gone to the E.R. at the hospital near the Hampton, our home, but his doctor wanted to see him personally. (I will finish this later after we return home—gotta go.)

It is now evening. James is dozing in his recliner, and I am resting on the sofa nearby. When we saw the doctor this morning, he did not hear anything in James' lungs to suggest Pneumonia but felt he had bronchitis and even the beginning of C.O.P.D. Because his blood oxygen level was low, the nurse gave James a breathing treatment, which gave almost immediate relief. Then the doctor sent us home with an electric compressor Nebulizer." He also gave us medication for inhalation treatments to be given twice a day for two weeks. We finished the first of twenty-eight treatments a short while ago. I discovered within thirty seconds that James could not remember to keep the mouthpiece in place. Therefore, I sat beside him for what seemed like an eternity until the medication was all gone. I have a very strong feeling that this is going to be a very long two weeks, requiring supernatural patience. Help me, Father. But James is worth it, and I will faithfully pray for patience. "I will be sending this text message to Heaven twice daily:

"Needed: Extra strength, patience, and endurance."

(in Building Two, The Hampton at Pearland)

(Lucy)

My Journal — August 3, 2011

"Father, as I serve James today doing the most menial, sometimes distasteful and unthinkable tasks, please help me to do these things as Christ would have done them—with unconditional love and patience. Help me to remember that James, in his total, childlike dependence on me, deserves my very best and all my love and patience.

We all have our "Giants" to face. You know mine. This terrible disease has ravaged James' mind and body for years. I'm daily fighting my "Giant"—Alzheimer's—with my faith and hope focused on You. I have no doubt that You give me all the strength and patience I need to endure each new challenge. Thank You, Father, for the lessons You are teaching me in this very difficult season." (Lucy)

My Journal — September 5, 2011

"Father, as You already know, some of my days are more difficult than others. These are the days when James is unusually confused and anxious. The last few days he has been fixated on one thing: "Going home."

All day he asks, "When can we go home"? I need to go home."
He gets very upset when I tell him, "We are home."

By the time I get him ready for bed, and he finally falls
asleep, I am exhausted, emotionally and physically. Today
in my spirit, I hear You say, "Remember Lucy when you
can't take another step, I will carry you. I will give you the
strength, energy and patience to endure whenever you ask
Me." And I know You will. Thank You Father.

Be with the children as they come to celebrate James' eighty-
fifth birthday today. I will be taking everyone out to dinner
this evening to one of our favorite restaurants. I am so glad
our children are coming from San Antonio. I need to discuss
with all three sons an important and difficult decision about
their Dad's future care. Keeping him with me in the new
house I had built in June of this year, even with help, is
not meeting his needs. I know you will give us wisdom and
direction for the next step." (Lucy)

~ Faith ~

✝ Faith is not an emotion. It is objective trust placed in a very real God.

✝ You can't network, strong-arm, or sweet-talk your way into heaven. Your faith is all that counts.

✝ Never be ashamed of your faith.

✝ Seek to know God and faith will follow.

✝ Faith does not demand miracles, but often accomplishes them.

✝ Strive to be a person of faith rather than fame.

✝ As you exercise your courage, exercise your faith.

✝ Looking back on what God has done for you strengthens your faith in the future.

God, our Father, has planted in our hearts a very special provision for our journey with Alzheimer's, the "seed of faith."

Faith is so incredible; it's difficult to define. The writer of the book of Hebrews describes it this way: "The fundamental fact of existence is that this trust in God, this faith, is the firm foundation under everything that makes life worth living" (Hebrews 11:1 *The Message*).

I love the way Max Lucado defines faith in Grace for the Moment:[16] "Faith is a desperate dive out of a sinking boat of human effort and a prayer that God will be there to pull us out of the water."

My definition of faith has been born out of a desperate need for God's help during these thirteen years we've been living with Alzheimer's. I see my faith as a deliberate departure from common sense to an honest, bold prayer for God to enter the difficult circumstances and adversities of my life—and the absolute trust that He will. Thankfully, I can say this with confidence because every day I see His handiwork in the big and small things in my life. I'm discovering that the greater my need, the greater His concern and the sweeter His provision of faith.

You already know that I love the analogy of life as a journey. I love the word picture of a traveler, a pilgrim on a journey through unfamiliar, uncharted territory. This life we're living with our loved one with Alzheimer's is a journey, and we must all walk our path. But we never walk alone. Our faithful Father is always with us. He will "never leave us or forsake us" (Hebrews 13:5).

You also know that I love the Psalms. I've spent hours reading them since we began our journey. Fifteen of the Psalms: Psalm 120 through Psalm 134, are "pilgrim songs" or "songs of ascents." They were written by David or one of the "worship leaders" to be sung by those

16   Max Lucado, Grace For The Moment, J. Countryman, a Division of Thomas Nelson, Nashville, Tennessee, 2000, 151.

making their annual pilgrimage from the low-country to Jerusalem. The exception is Psalm 127, written by Solomon. I love them all, especially Psalm 121.

In *Psalm 121*, we can hear the psalmist calling out, "Lord I need your strength, help and protection on this journey." Those were my words eleven years ago. I felt lost in the wilderness of the dementia that day-by-day was robbing me of my husband, my traveling companion. I knew I couldn't handle what I was facing without God's help. As usual, my never-failing Father provided help in a very practical way. I wrote about this in my journal.

❧

My Journal — September 10, 2002

"James is reading the paper while I am writing this morning. Occasionally he will interrupt me to ask me what a certain word means. This morning it is "genetics." Yesterday, it was "sanctions." In dismay, I watch as his brilliant mind is slowly but surely slipping away almost like sand through an hourglass. I want desperately to stop the "grains of sand", but I can't. All I can do is to cry out to God for His help, which I do, frequently. He never lets me down.

A perfect example of God's constant concern for me is His pointing out a certain book I picked up last week at a Christian bookstore. I was looking for something to read on a bus trip James and I are taking with friends in a few weeks. I picked up this particular book because it was written by one of my favorite authors, David Jeremiah. The title of the book, When Your World Falls Apart, had called out to me at the bookstore that day. I purchased it, along with several others, planning to pack them for our trip. I couldn't wait to read this book, and I've been devouring it every chance I get.

The book is Dr. Jeremiah's story about his totally unexpected diagnosis of Lymphoma in 1994. He refers to this as his "bend in the road." He talks about the fact that life can be so normal and our future so secure, and then suddenly our road takes an unexpected turn. (I can certainly testify to the truth of that statement). I am amazed at how closely his reaction and emotions to his "bend in the road" parallel my reaction to James' diagnosis—Alzheimer's. I have no doubt in my mind that God has placed this book in my hands to help strengthen me for what is ahead on our journey with dementia.

Thank you, Father, for this book and its author and for all the ways you bless me when I place my faith and trust in you." (Lucy)

As I continued to read David Jeremiah's book, I was amazed that he, too, loves the word picture of a pilgrim on a journey. Equally astonishing is that he also loves Psalm 121 and devoted the entire third chapter to this Psalm. He says this about it: "The psalmist lifts his eyes to the hills above and sees the One who is not only the destination of the journey, but also the strength for every step of it." He adds, "He is never too great to care; we are never too small for His caring. The Psalm reflects on a God who soothes us in our anxiety and watches over us as a shepherd with his sheep."[17]

When your journey brought you to your "bend in the road," your "disruptive moment," you must have felt lost as I did. You were probably filled with an unaccustomed sense of helplessness. Perhaps you cried out, as I did, "Father, I need your help."

It is my prayer that you have discovered that the One who created and sustained every atom of the Universe can sustain you. There will be times, as we continue our journey into the unknown when we will have moments of deep anxiety. In those times, we must remember to take a deep breath, let it out slowly and, in faith, look at our Guide, our faithful God. These are the things we can know for sure that He will do for us:

---

17   David Jeremiah, *When Your World Falls Apart*, Thomas Nelson (Word Publishing), Nashville, Tennessee, 2000, 59.

✝ He will see us.

✝ He will never keep us waiting.

✝ He never sleeps.

✝ He's never out of town.

✝ His "cell phone" is always on, therefore He is never out of reach.

✝ He will watch over us and protect us. He is our "Security System"

My Journal — June 10, 2008

"I'm here at my Bethel after an exhausting night. James got up during the night but did not make it to the bathroom. He got as far as the foot of our four-poster bed, where he made a puddle on the wood floor. Before I could get to him, he stepped in the puddle, slipped and fell, bumping his left hip and shoulder on the bedpost. After I cleaned up the urine with a large towel, I finally got him up. I'm pretty sure his "angel" was standing by, ready to help. I bathed him, put dry clothes on him, checked his bruises, and got him back into bed. I then finished mopping and cleaning the floor, washed my hands and climb wearily back into bed. It was 3:19 A.M. James reached over and stroked my arm. He said, "Are you okay? Did you hurt yourself?" I didn't know whether to laugh or to strangle him. He is so precious, and I love him so much. But there are times I can't help wondering "Lord, how long?"

My faith is all that sustains. Even though life gave us what I prayed would never happen, I know that I can trust God with the future, knowing that He loves us and will be walking by our side forever. That means all the way to eternity with Him. And that is the goal of our faith.

It seems that the greater my needs, the bolder and more sincere my prayers have become. Someone said recently "God honors bold prayers because bold prayers honor God." I love that. I believe that faith is my most valuable asset. I've heard Dr. Charles Stanley say that, and I agree. Also, I think that God is using this tragedy, Alzheimer's, to develop in me a stronger, more mature faith. Soon after our journey began, I realized that, until tested, my faith had been naïve.

Daily, here on my knees at my Bethel, I'm discovering a deeper faith and finding more intimacy with my Heavenly Father.

For those things, I am very thankful." (Lucy)

My Journal — June 11, 2008

I'm here at my Bethel this morning, tired but grateful for another day. James and I are not sleeping much, and I am exhausted. James sleeps a lot during the day, but I never do. There are too many things to do, and I'm having trouble, even now, letting go of my 'perfectionism'. I'm asking God to help me to let go of some things and trust Him more.

I want so much for my testimony to encourage those who are watching to see how I'm dealing with this tragedy. I want them to see, lived out in my daily walk, my faith and trust in God's faithfulness and love. I realize that how I respond to our difficulties and trials will affect those watching my life. I want them to know that the faith I've talked about, sung about and taught about all these years is real. When they look at my life, I want them to see someone who relies wholly on her Heavenly Father for strength and courage.

I don't want to waste my pain. I want my testimony to glorify God and to point others to Him." (Lucy)

I know we can always trust God who, in contrast to the world, has no history of failure. Also, I know that God has called me to the "ministry" of caring for my sweet James. Concerning this call, I will say along with Paul: "I have no regrets. I couldn't be surer of my ground. The One I've trusted in can take care of what He's trusted me to do to the end" (2 Timothy 1:12 *The Message*).

By faith, we can take our fears, our worries, our sadness, our anxiety, our exhaustion to God, the One Who is immovable and unchangeable. When we do this, He will faithfully meet every need, proving that our faith is of "greater worth than gold" (1 Peter 1:7).

Facing tragedy or life storms of any kind can be extremely difficult. But in the midst of heartache and pain, we can find the hope and courage to go on. With God's help, the help of caring family members and friends, and the encouragement found in the Bible and other resources, we will receive the necessary strength to overcome.

You may be thinking, "I don't know how I can ever get through this." Or you may be battling powerful feelings of despair, suffering, confusion, fear, worry, and even anger. These are all normal responses to this nightmare we call Alzheimer's.

But as difficult as this nightmare may be, we are not alone. God is with us always. He loves us and cares about what is going on in our life. He hears our cries and sees our pain. Moreover, He understands.

My Journal — March 3, 2009

"Last night, the wind blew very hard and turned over a chair on the deck outside our bedroom. The noise woke me, and for a moment, I was frightened, not knowing what had happened. James, who never sleeps soundly, was also awake and frightened. He kept saying, "What was that noise? Are we safe? Are you sure? How do you know?" I wanted James to hold me as he had always done when I had a bad dream or was frightened by an unidentified noise. Instead, I got out of bed, checked to find the source of the sound, and then got back into bed. I held James close and reassured him that we were okay, that he was safe. It was 1:48 A.M. After he finally went back to sleep, I stayed awake, grieving for what is forever lost.

Again, I was reminded that, for the rest of his life, I will be the "Mother", and he will be my "little man." I am so grateful that, through faith, I am shielded by God's power, though for a little while I may have to suffer grief in all kinds of trials. [My Paraphrase of 1 Peter 1:5-6]

Father, thank You that what started as a sleep-deprived morning has become a time of praise and worship." (Lucy)

My Journal — March 28, 2010

"Last night, at this time, I thought I had finished the chapter on "Faith", but God was not finished. He knew what was coming. One of my favorite descriptions of faith is this:

"Faith begins when you see God on the mountain

and you are in the valley, and you know

you're too weak to make the climb.

You see what you need, you

see what you have, and

what you have isn't enough

to accomplish anything."

Max Lucado[18]

That's where I am today: faced with the painful, monumental decision to sell my beautiful "miracle house" on Rainbow Bend Drive. It is filled with things I have carefully and joyfully collected through the years—things that I love. They are treasures and memories that are part of who I am: Mother's and Grandmother's blue and white china; Independence Ironstone I received as a wedding gift; dozens of teapots; tiny blue tea sets; blue Spode plates and lamps; blue quilts and linens and pillows; cobalt bottles I have collected over the past forty-three years; dozens of cookbooks; clocks; Precious Moments figurines and pieces of crystal (gifts from my sons); Depression glass pieces and luncheon sets; pictures; Mother's paintings; tablecloths, napkins, placemats, chargers—all with centerpieces to match; Christmas china and decorative pieces of all kinds, lots of seasonal decorations; hundreds of books; and wonderful furniture pieces. I could go on and on.

How do I decide what I can keep and what I must share with others, hoping that somehow they will come to love and cherish them as I do?

The plan is for us to sell our home and move into a Brookdale Community, the Hampton at Pearland, an Assisted Living Complex with an award winning Memory Care facility on the grounds. The director has generously offered to create

---

18   *GRACE for the Moment*, p. 291.

for us a large, two-room apartment from two one-room apartments. Even so, we will be moving from a large four-bedroom home with lots of storage (and a two car garage). This will require the most brilliant, efficient downsizing in history.

As painful as all of this is, I will remember that James and his happiness, safety, and welfare are so much more important than "things"—no matter what they are. After God, James is my most precious treasure. "Things" will someday pass away, but my love and devotion to James and God will last forever. Although what God is asking me to do seems confusing and, at times, even unreasonable, in faith I will trust Him.

I worry that I'm not up to this task, emotionally or physically. I feel somehow 'trapped' and fearful, not knowing how all the pieces of this puzzle will fit together. It has been eleven years since we began this journey—this "faith journey." It is time.

I know in my heart that my only hope is putting all my faith in my Father in heaven. I'm asking Him today for supernatural strength and a miracle. God already knows my limitations, and I already know His strength, power, and faithfulness. Together we will do this—God and I." (Lucy)

I wrote this journal entry three and a half years ago. During these years, God has been even more faithful than I could have imagined. I once read a statement about faith which is so appropriate here:

"Faith does not demand miracles, but often accomplishes them." I could not have said it better. But I can say, "Amen."

~ Grace ~

"Grace is God's best idea. His decision to ravage a people by love, to rescue passionately, and to restore justly. What rivals it? Of all his wondrous works, grace is the magnum opus."~Max Lucado[19]

---

19   GRACE: More Than We Deserve, Greater Than We Imagine by Max Lucado, (2012)

Truth We Know About Grace

- ✝ It is amazing.
- ✝ It is always available.
- ✝ It is empowering.
- ✝ It is extreme.
- ✝ It is gracious.
- ✝ It is greater than our sins.
- ✝ It is intentional.
- ✝ It is life-saving, eternally.
- ✝ It is merciful.
- ✝ It is perfect.
- ✝ It is powerful.
- ✝ It is shocking.
- ✝ It is supernatural.
- ✝ It is transforming.
- ✝ It is unexpected.
- ✝ It is unmerited.

Two Quotes I Love:

"God's grace is a come-as-you are promise from a
One-Of-A-Kind King."
~Max Lucado (*Grace for the Moment* – May 18)

"Grace goes first. 'While we were still sinners, Christ died for us'
(Romans 5:8). Jesus went first. Grace says, 'I'm not gonna wait;
I'm not gonna meet you in the middle. I'm just gonna go first.'"
~Andy Stanley (*In Touch*, interview about his book
The Grace of God), *In Touch* magazine, January 2011, p. 16-19.

Were it not for God's provision of grace, I would not be writing these words, and you would not be reading them. Grace was given to us through Jesus before the beginning of time—God's gift from start to finish.

Grace is so amazing, so shocking, so outrageous, it's hard to wrap our finite mind around it. It's like trying to hold smoke, or a cloud, or a moonbeam in your hand.

Grace is God standing between us and our need and His waiting to meet that need—not too early, not too late, but at precisely the right time. The Bible tells us this: "Let us then fearlessly and confidently and boldly draw near to the throne of grace—the throne of God's unmerited favor (to us sinners); that we may receive mercy (for our failures) and find grace to help in good time for every need—appropriate help and well-timed help, coming just when we need it" (Hebrews 5:16, AMP).

No one who ever turned to God for help was disappointed by His response. We must never be too proud to ask for His help, His grace. We need to realize that God's grace is extreme. It nailed Jesus, His only Son, to a cruel cross as a sacrifice for the sins of mankind. That is the "point" of grace. Grace is God's riches and forgiveness lavished on those of us who, only moments before, stood accused.

My "moment of grace" came in a College dorm room in January of 1954 at a time in my life when I had lost direction; when I was questioning the validity of all I had been taught and had been living out in my life until that moment. On my knees, in a simple, sincere prayer, I asked Jesus to come into my heart, forgive my sins and give me a new beginning. I got up from my knees, instantly and forever changed. In that moment of grace, I was given a new life, an eternal life in heaven. It was a turning point in my life and the beginning of a future filled with hope and purpose. Never again would I question my salvation, this wonderful grace, accepted by faith into my heart.

Just as the scripture verse Hebrews 5:16 promises, since that day, God has provided for my every need with well-timed help, just when I've needed it. Later on in this chapter, I share some of the ways God has provided His 'well-timed help' on our journey with Alzheimer's.

God has so many goals for us as Christians, but sometimes it's hard to understand this when our situation seems too painful to bear.

But the promise that God gave Paul when he thought his pain was too much to bear applies to us today: "My grace is sufficient for you" (2 Corinthians 12:9). You may be asking, "But how does this grace work out in my everyday life as I deal with the difficulties of caring for my loved one with dementia?"

In a devotional in *In Touch,* November 17, 2011, Dr. Charles Stanley addresses this very appropriate question:

✝ "The Lord's grace releases His supernatural power within us so we can endure life's hardships with a godly attitude.

✝ Grace builds our confidence in the sovereign Lord. Nothing looks hopeless when we focus on Him.

✝ We discover the assurance of God's sustaining presence as He walks with us every step of the way.

✝ Because we experience His care for us, we can show empathy and love to others facing hard times.

✝ During fiery trails, grace works to transform our character so that others can see Jesus reflected in us."

Difficulties on our journey as caregivers are unavoidable. That's why we need to claim God's grace if we are to walk successfully through our trials. No matter how agonizing they are, we can look ahead with confidence at the goal before us: "keeping the faith, finishing well." It is only when we rely on our strength and wisdom that the obstacles ahead seem insurmountable, leaving us discouraged and ready to give up.

My Journal — January 2, 2009

I'm reminiscing today about the year that has just passed. As James' Alzheimer's advanced, he and I became "homebound" by the end of 2007. Because of this, I found myself in a private storm of weariness and loneliness. Also, I discovered something about myself. I had been maintaining my image of Super Wife, Super Mom, Super Strong Christian for so long, I had difficulty admitting to others that I needed help. I had always been the strong one giving others help. I didn't even know how to express my emotions. I was hesitant to share my anxieties and despair with anyone, even my family and fellow Christian friends, for fear they would think that my faith was weak.

In my desperation, I turned more and more to God. Although I had served Him faithfully for years, I found myself longing for a deeper, more intimate relationship with Him. As I reached out to God, I discovered that He was even more eager than I to share such a relationship—one that would fill my loneliness with His love and grace.

In my daily quiet times with Him, through prayer and Bible study, God revealed to me a startling truth. He pointed out that, for years, I had been running the wrong "race." Rather than relying wholly on His grace, I had too often been relying on my strength, talents, and skills. The truths I discovered in the many hours I spent with God the Father were priceless. As I listened to Him speak personally to me through scriptures, many already familiar and well loved, I experienced a new level of understanding of His grace.

As I received the comfort and encouragement I so desperately needed, I began to feel a real burden to share with others this priceless treasure of grace I had discovered. I especially wanted to share with other caregivers that they, too, could experience this great "treasure trove of grace." Grace that was the answer to all my needs; grace that allowed me to lay everything in my life before God with no apology or hesitation, knowing that His love and grace would cover it all.

This burden that I felt last year to share what God was doing in the midst of my "drudgery filled" life was the motivation and inspiration for the book I began writing. I didn't want to hoard any part of the treasure of grace I had found. I can't resist quoting David Jeremiah's definition of grace found in his book, Captured by Grace. He says, "Grace is the delivery of a jewel that nobody ordered, a burst of light in a room where everyone forgot it was dark."[20] He writes these words following a story he tells about an amazing example of grace lived out in our present day world. It's a story that warms the heart. The tragedy is that after we are touched for a moment, many will go right back to their struggle-filled lives. But not everyone. Not I. I'm again borrowing inspiration from Dr. Jeremiah's words. For me, the discovery of grace was "like finding a knot hole in the high gates of heaven." I couldn't tear myself away from peeping through it. And I was left to "wonder why, if this thing called grace is so magnificent —and if it is a standard option for every moment—why is it so rare and isolated?"[21] It was this very question, so graphically stated by Dr. Jeremiah, that created deep within me an urgency to call others, especially fellow caregivers, "to the knot hole."

Thus, the conception of this book took place, the seed placed there by my awe of God's great treasure, "grace." I will, with God's help, continue to write our story—God's story—until it is finished." (Lucy)

It is God's love that continues to provide the grace needed for our faith journey with Alzheimer's. Someone has said, "Without the burden of pain and suffering, it is impossible to reach the height of grace because the gift of grace increases as our struggle increases.[22] The most comforting thing is that, by grace, God takes us "as is", with all our mess-ups, imperfections, and failures. Because He is our Father, we don't need to be 'perfect' for Him to love us. We never need to "negotiate." His grace, His unmerited favor, stands between us and whatever it is we are

---

20   David Jeremiah, *Captured by Grace: No One is Beyond the Reach of a Loving God,*(Nashville: Integrity Publishers, 2006).

21   Ibid, 13

22   St. Rose of Lima (1586-1617)

facing. If we truly desire to be the faithful, loving caregiver that God has called us to be, we will see every trial and challenge as an opportunity to demonstrate that His grace really is "sufficient for every need" (2 Corinthians 12:9). Even though God may not remove our "thorn", Alzheimer's, He has promised that on this journey we are never at the mercy of the unknowns ahead.

Psalm 84 tells us that, as each traveler on his way to "Zion" passes through his "valleys", God's with him. Along with the psalmist, we can be confident of victory, no matter how high our mountains or how long and rough our valleys. This is because all of our traveling needs have been provided by the Master Guide. That's grace.

My Journal — February 10, 2010

This morning I'm at my Bethel after a troubled night. It has become very apparent that I can no longer care for James and all of his needs without help. I am faced with this reality even though I can scarcely bear the thought of what this may involve. Lately, I'm feeling lost and overwhelmed. There are so many decisions to be made in the near future—decisions I can only make with God's wisdom and guidance.

As I kneel here, asking for His peace and direction, God is reminding me that I can move forward in the days ahead, safe in the realization that nothing I am facing can ever put me beyond the reach of His grace. I pick up my Bible and turn instinctively to the passage that has been my 'lifeline' for the past eight years, Romans 8:28. I read it aloud, "And we know that in all things God works for the good of those who love him, who have been called according to his purpose." I read it again, and the words "all things" seem to echo in the room and my heart. I notice that in the margin of my Bible I have written these words: "This verse is my best friend; it is engraved on my heart by the finger of God Himself." Beside them is the date: December 9, 2007. I realize that this was when I knew I could never again leave James home alone.

Today I will remember that "all things" means All Things. I know that whatever God chooses will be better than anything I could choose on my own. When I feel overwhelmed, I will say, "God always does all things well." (Lucy)

My Journal — April 19, 2010

I'm up very early, and I'm reading my journal entry from February 10, 2010. I'm thinking about how frustrating it can be, when I'm struggling with heartache and exhaustion, for someone to glibly quote Bible verses and spiritual cliché to me. Someone said to me shortly after James was diagnosed with Alzheimer's, "If your faith were strong enough, James would be healed." I'm writing this today to emphasize that I never want to leave the impression that I am "over spiritualizing" my pain. On the other hand, I never want to "water down" God's amazing grace and power in the midst of my pain and heartache. I want my words to be more than a "feel good" devotional. Rather, I want them to address the nitty-gritty reality of what we're dealing with on a daily basis. More than anything, I want them to reveal a "hands on" Father who understands everything about us.

When God said to Paul in 2 Corinthians 12:9: "My grace is sufficient for you, for my power is made perfect in weakness," He wasn't giving him some trite "religious" platitude. He was giving Paul (and us) a promise of hope through His personal intervention in our time of weakness and suffering. As illogical as it seems, God is promising His presence in our circumstances, changing our suffering and weakness into a blessing. I'll remember His promise as I deal with the physical and emotional stress of this move to the Hampton.

"Father, I need all of your power available to me today."
(Lucy)

You may remember that, at the beginning of this chapter, I said I would share some of the ways God has provided well-timed help during our journey. On the very day that I wrote the journal entry you just read, God showed up to affirm that He was present in my circumstances that day. I took a break from packing to walk down the sidewalk to our mailbox. In the mail was the May 2010 *In Touch* magazine from the Charles Stanley Ministry. I could scarcely wait to open it. God never fails to speak words of encouragement to me through the articles and devotionals contained there. Although I didn't really have time, I sat down, propped up my tired feet and opened it to page thirty. There at the top of the page, in large print, were the words, "My grace is sufficient for you, for my power is made perfect in weakness." I was stunned. I knew that God was personally sending me a message that He knew I needed His strength that day. I have no idea who wrote the article. I only saved the one page but I want to share some of it with you: "God is speaking about personal, private pain that no one on earth can experience with you or for you or completely understand, simply because they're not you. His power dwelling in and springing from your weakness isn't just about helping you hang in there and survive. It's about His grace completing its effect in your life. This is reality: that the Creator is literally speaking His story into yours—that He has entered into the pain you are otherwise alone in and has borne it for you on His own back, carrying you, as you really can't carry it alone."

The author of these words had no idea when he or she wrote them that they would speak such strength and peace and encouragement into my exhausted body and broken heart that very day. It was God's well-timed help.

My Journal —May 10, 2010

I'm writing this morning from my new "Bethel" at the Hampton. I haven't written much since my last journal entry on April 19, 2010. The last two weeks of April were probably the most difficult ones of my life, physically and emotionally. When the decision was made, after much prayer, to sell our large home and move into a two-room apartment at the Hampton at Pearland, I knew nothing would be easy. But I knew that God would be with me. I watched in amazement as He miraculously and dramatically showed up, time after time—not too early, not too late, but just in time. When I was utterly exhausted, I just let Him take over.

I discovered that God the Father was making sure that I had what I needed, just when I needed it. My sons had used a small moving company in the past and knew the owners personally. I called them, and they were awesome. Three of our bedrooms had carpet, and once the furniture was moved out, I was stressed by the carpet's condition. The young movers spoke up and said, "We also clean carpets." (Which they did, superbly.) Just before they returned with their carpet cleaning equipment, a woman and her daughter came to pick up a desk they had purchased earlier at my garage sale. I said to them, "You don't by any chance know someone who cleans houses, do you?" They laughed and said, "That's what we do." Actually, they also regularly cleaned a nearby church. They left, promising to return early the next morning with their cleaning supplies.

I was so relieved because I had just learned from my Realtor that the closing date for my house had been moved up two days. I knew there was no way, even if I worked all night, that I could clean the entire house, now that it was empty.

By now, James and I were moved into our new apartment. I left our now "almost vacant" home each evening, just in time to arrive at the Hampton before dark. I picked up James at Clare Bridge where he stayed during the day, walked next door to our building, got him ready for bed, then collapsed, only to start the same routine early the next day.

I met my cleaning ladies, my "angels" at the house very early the next morning. Never in my life have I witnessed such thoroughness, such professionalism, such precision. They started in the master closet, worked their way through the master bath and bedroom, down the hall, and throughout the rest of the house, cleaning everything in their path to perfection.

When they were finished, my house looked like a new house. I sent them home with a huge box filled with seasonal wreaths, flower arrangements, shoes and purses and anything else that was left in the house. The only thing left was a recliner sitting on the deck and a large skateboard ramp left in the driveway. As I was deliberating about what to do with them since the final walk-through with the buyers and their Realtor was later that day, the doorbell rang. A man, in broken English, asked if he could have the things stacked at the curb for the heavy trash pick-up. I said, "Yes, take it all and would you like a recliner?" He said "Si" and moved it from the deck to his truck.

By now, nothing would have surprised me. I walked down the front sidewalk to the driveway wondering what in the world I could do with an enormous, but thankfully on wheels, skateboard ramp. As I was standing there looking at it, a young man came across the street from a house two doors down. He said, "What are you going to do with the ramp?" I said, "Give it to you if you want it." He said, "Are you serious?" He then effortlessly pushed it across the street, thanking me profusely. And I was thanking God profusely for His amazing grace.

God Himself had worked out all the details, not too early, not too late, just in time. This, dear friends, is the reality of God's grace applied to our everyday lives. "Father, as I'm resting and recovering from our move to the Hampton, there are no words to fully express my gratitude for Your love and grace. I will share my experiences and blessings with everyone I encounter today." (Lucy)

My Journal —October 10, 2010

"I'm writing today on the upstairs deck of my building at the Hampton. It's Sunday, and I just walked James next door to Clare Bridge, the Memory Care facility where he spends each day. We had a restless night, and I let him sleep a little later than usual. I'm taking a break from teaching the early morning Bible Study class I've taught for over ten years. With winter coming, I worry about getting there on time in case of bad weather.

It is a wonderful fall day, and I'm experiencing a sweet sense of God's love and grace. The sky is a beautiful blue sea filled with fluffy, white cotton "islands." The only movement is a tiny, silver jet plane crossing the expanse of blue and disappearing into a cloud. I'm so aware at this moment of God's presence in this beautiful tabernacle of nature. I'm also aware that, according to scripture, He is looking down from above, aware of me and my needs. He knows that there are times when this "new normal" doesn't feel normal at all. Sometimes I am so very lonely for the familiarity of my home and the friends I left behind. It's humbling to know that during this time, the Creator and Sustainer of all this incredible beauty cares about me. He knows my "imperfect" self so well and loves me anyway—that's grace.

Today, in this "tabernacle" of His creation, I will worship Him, thank Him, and praise His name in my own private worship center, the sanctuary in my heart, God's dwelling place.

I'm just sitting out here, soaking up all this beauty, all this peace flowing from God's supply of grace for me. Jesus could always see His Father's supply. That is my heart's desire. I'm already thanking God in advance for the grace I know He will continue to provide, at the exact time I will need it. Just as Jesus is always in the Father's presence, so am I. I want to live with the "rhythm of God's presence constantly playing in my heart." (Lucy)

A decade after James' diagnosis I am still experiencing the same grace which covered me that day in July of 1999. Occasionally, I open my Bible and read 2 Corinthians 12. Each time I do, I realize once more that our trials are allowed by God to help us keep in touch with our limitations and to enable us to grow spiritually. Sometimes, I wonder what I would have been like had I not encountered "my thorn", the adversity connected with caring for James. Would I know the power of God grace? Would I experience the joy of the sweet intimacy that I share with my Father? Would I have the strength I've discovered as I've dealt with every painful, difficult situation? Would I have the faith I'll need as I face the unknown future? Would I have the assurance I now possess to know that, no matter how much longer the journey will be or how it will end, God's grace will be sufficient?

I can say with confidence that the answer to all of the above is "no, I would not" – And I can say, "thank you, Father, for everything that you have taught me."

~ Hope ~

Hope is invaluable. Everyone needs hope. God, our Father, knew this when He packed this provision for our journey with Alzheimer's. He knows that hope is fundamental to our faith in Him.

I love Hebrews 11:1 which tells us, "Now faith is being sure of what we hope for and certain of what we do not see." All of us have hopes and dreams and, as Christians, we have every reason to be hopeful. After all, God is good. He loves us, and He has given us everything we need — most importantly, the priceless gift of eternal life with Him. Even though we believe this, during our dark, difficult days on this journey, it's easy to lose sight of hope.

I remember that during the early days of our journey, James and I held tightly to hope. We prayed that we would wake up and discover this was just a bad dream; we prayed that perhaps the diagnosis was wrong; we prayed for miraculous healing for James' brain. Ultimately, we were forced to accept the reality and truth of our situation. We also would come to realize that "The Lord is good, a refuge in time of trouble. He cares for those who trust in Him" (Nahum 1:7). He is the one who knows our every need.

As the weeks and months passed, we learned that Jesus is the reason for and the source of our hope. We developed a deeper, more personal awareness of His presence, and we were confident that He was walking this new path with us. Knowing that this journey was taking us into frightening, unfamiliar territory, I found indescribable comfort and hope in His presence. Not knowing where we were going or how long this journey would take, I turned to God's word for answers.

By God's grace, I found the hope I was seeking in His Word. As I opened my Bible each morning, God poured promise after promise out of His Word, planting seeds of hope deep in my heart. He showed me these verses (and many others):

✝ 2 Thessalonians 2:16, "May our Lord Jesus Christ himself and God our Father, who loved us and by his grace gave us eternal encouragement and good hope, encourage your hearts."

✝ Genesis 18:14, "Is anything too hard for God?"

✝ Hebrews 13:5-6, "Never will I leave you, never will I forsake you. So we say with confidence, 'The Lord is my helper; I will not be afraid.' "

✝ Micah 7:7, "But as for me, I watch in hope for the Lord, I wait for God my Savior; my God will hear me."

✝ Psalm 119:49, "Remember your word to your servant, for you have given me hope."

✝ Psalm 42:5, "Why are you downcast, 0 my soul? Why so disturbed within me? Put your hope in God, for I will yet praise him, my Savior and my God."

✝ Romans 5:5, "Hope does not disappoint us because God has poured out his love into our hearts by the Holy Spirit, whom he has given us."

In these scriptures I found endless and relentless hope and encouragement and a balm for my wounded heart. These verses said to me, "No matter how dim the path or treacherous the trail, don't give up, no matter how much you want to." They revealed to me that hope is not just an optimistic wish. It is the perfect confidence that God will fulfill all his promises to us. Every day God reminds me, "My grace is sufficient for you, Lucy, for my power is made perfect in your weakness"(2 Corinthians 12:9, paraphrased).

That memorable day in July of 1999, James and I encountered a large obstacle, an enormous obstruction on our typically straight, smooth path. The diagnosis that day was "a gut-wrenching moment, a life changing event." As James and I discussed our feelings, we talked about others, friends and family, who had experienced similar moments in their lives. We knew that many of them had faced with great courage and dignity their dreaded diagnosis: "Cancer", "MS", "Diabetes", "Brain tumor", "Alzheimer's." We wanted to exhibit the same kind of courage and faith they had shown. We wanted to be able to say, "Father, you are so good, and we know you love us. Thank you for this trial, this 'prison' of Alzheimer's that holds us captive. We know that you have a purpose for even this." God has told us in his Word in 1 Thessalonians 5:18, to be thankful for everything, in all circumstances, and James and I have always tried to be obedient. In all honesty, though, could we really be thankful for the trials that we knew were ahead on this journey? Could we actually find the kind of faith and hope that this required?

We found the answer in God's Word in Romans 5:2-5: "...we rejoice in the hope of the glory of God. And not only that, but we rejoice in our sufferings, knowing that suffering produces endurance, and endurance produces character, and character produces hope, and hope does not put us to shame, because God's love has been poured into our hearts through the Holy Spirit who has been given to us" (ESV).

Now, when my hope starts to waver, I look back and remember God's faithfulness in the difficult times and how I survived and emerged unscathed and stronger. Recalling past victories helps me to have hope for tomorrow in spite of the challenges on my path today. I will remember that as long as I have hope, no night will be completely dark, and I can find joy even when my heart is breaking.

I want my hope to reflect my faith in God. I want it to be a testimony to my belief that this part of our journey has meaning and purpose even though I often experience times of grief and anxiety. I realize that hope is not a possession; I don't own it. It's an attitude, a way of living, of being. As James' caregiver, it's finding meaning in a gentle touch and kiss, snuggling together on "our love seat", holding hands, singing the old hymns of faith that James loves. It's in calm, patient conversation, loving looks, looking at pictures and recalling and discussing happy memories. It's in my constant reassurance of my love for him and the promise that I will never forget him or abandon him. It's in James' declaration of his love for me every day: "I love you with all my heart." and "You're too wonderful to be real." It's in his reminder every night, "Till death do us part," something he never forgets even when he doesn't know who or where he is.

These Are The Facts I Believe About Hope

- In January of 1954, God the Father, in his great mercy gave me "new birth into a living hope through the resurrection of Jesus Christ from the dead" (1 Peter 1:3). That living hope has sustained me every day of the past fifty-nine years.

- For the person who has no hope, life looks like a long, dark tunnel going nowhere. Without hope, that's how my life would have looked that day, July 22, 1999. That's when the word "Alzheimer's" would become a daily part of my life and my vocabulary for the next thirteen years.

- My personal relationship with Jesus gives me a hope that is an anchor for my soul. This anchor, which represents safety and security in my life, holds me firm in the storms that are an inevitable part of our life with Alzheimer's.

- Prevailing hope keeps me healthy—emotionally, physically, and mentally. Proverbs 13:12 tells us: "Hope deferred makes the heart sick, but a longing fulfilled is a tree of life." Hope can help us to look ahead with the assurance of a better tomorrow.

- My hope stands firm on God's promises in His Word, promises He always keeps. His Word tells me that He always wants what's best for His children. God is our hope for the future. As I look into the unknowns ahead, with no clear path to follow, I must confess that I am sometimes afraid, even though I know that He is waiting there in my future, giving me hope.

- The Apostle Paul tells us in Philippians 4:19, "My God will meet all your needs according to His glorious riches in Christ Jesus." This doesn't say that He may or that He is able; it says, "He will." Therefore, even when the thing I hope for doesn't happen, I can know without a doubt that it was not in His will for me. I know that somewhere further down the path, He has something much better than I can even imagine.

- Fellow caregivers of Alzheimer's sufferers, we can find hope in caregiving. I believe, however, that our hope must be directed toward what is possible, not what we fantasize will happen. Although our hope may not free us from hardships and heartaches, with hope we can claim God's promise of a brighter tomorrow. Our hope can also help us to be grateful for each day with our loved one.

- Setbacks and losses can occur quickly and intensely, and sometimes it's impossible to find meaning or any promise of relief. Despite this, we are not without hope. The very fact that we persevere is an intense and profound declaration that we have not turned our back on hope. Because our hope is anchored in Jesus, when we are at our wits end, we can call out the name—"Jesus"—and we will find in Him the hope and help that we need.

My Journal — September 8, 2012

Today James and I have entered our last season together, the "Hospice Season." Father, thank You that even though I may temporarily find myself in a place of hopelessness and enormous emotional pain, I can know that your hope is always available. I read somewhere that hope is the power that gives us the power to step into an uncertain future, shape it, and infuse it with meaning. With You, Father, I can recognize that today is only a moment in a longer life of meaningful experiences and relationships.

Your Word tells us that "no matter what the future holds for us, we can have hope that we are anchored to a firm foundation that can never be shaken" (my paraphrase of Isaiah 28:16). I'm going to make every effort to be hope-filled, even when my situation seems to say, "all is lost." I'm claiming the reality of Your unconditional love as the reason for my hope, even though James and I have entered this "new season."

Father, You know that I want to be a catalyst of hope for all who may need it. I want to leave the evidence of my hope everywhere I go—to share that hope is the "life-jacket" that has brought me safely to this point in my journey. I want to tell everyone who asks that Your gift of hope has kept me afloat when I thought my heart would break; when my world was falling apart; when I watched my dreams crumble; when I became the mother to James, "my little man." Thank You for giving me hope today." (Lucy)

When we need answers, we look to the authorities who specialize in our particular problem. There were two women who I consider specialists in the field of dispensing hope in the midst of severe heartache. One of them was Catherine Marshall, whose husband Peter Marshall, while serving as Chaplain to the United States Senate, died of a sudden massive heart attack. Out of her pain and heartache came several books, the best known, *A Man Called Peter*. In one of my journals, I have a quote from her, "God is the only one who can make the valley of trouble a door of hope." Even after her death in 1983, her legacy of faith and hope in the face of adversity lives on.

The other "specialist" in painful matters of the heart was Barbara Johnson, one of the Women of Faith speakers and one of my favorite authors. She was an authority on hope, having lost two of her three sons who died in their twenties. One was killed in action in Vietnam; one tragically killed by a drunk driver. Her third and youngest son, who is gay, was estranged from her for twelve years. I hang on for dear life to every word she so eloquently shared in her writings.

One of her quotes from *Boundless Love*[23] is included in my journal, dated November 1, 2001: "God believes in you, therefore your situation is never hopeless." That was timely encouragement for me in those early years of our journey.

This is my sincere offer to you: to share with you everything God has taught me and gifted me with during my thirteen years as caregiver to the dearest, most adorable, sweetest, handsomest and most godly man I've ever known: my husband and sweetheart, James Dishongh. I have, during these years, built up a very large bank account of comfort, courage, faith, joy, peace, hope, and strength. When your supply of these runs low, please feel free to borrow from my experiences and lessons gained from years of walking my path with Alzheimer's.

I'm writing these words on the second anniversary of James' death. I want you to feel free to call me, text me, write me, visit me, meet me for coffee. (I'll be the tiny little lady with white hair, wrinkles, and a twinkle in her eye.)

---

23   Women of Faith, *Boundless Love* (Zondervan Publishing House, Grand Rapids, Michigan, 2001); 126.

In the meantime, "our greatest hope as caregivers, formal or informal, is to be generators and vessels of love. Because in the end, love is all that matters and hope springs eternally out of love." [24]

"May the God of all hope fill you
with joy and peace"
(Romans 15:13).

~ Invitation to Journey with Jesus ~

If you were to stop a dozen people on the street and ask them, "What is your greatest need?" you'd probably get a dozen different answers.

If you were asked to name your greatest need as caregiver to your loved one with dementia, what would be your answer?

Without hesitation, I can tell you my greatest need as I care for my husband with Alzheimer's disease. I need a surrogate:

- Someone to step in and take my place when I desperately need another hour of sleep;

- Someone to worry for me so my mind can rest;

- Someone to experience my nagging frustrations and anxieties for an hour or two;

- Someone to be the caregiver to James so that I can take a long, soothing bubble bath without worrying about his safety;

24   Lela Knox Shanks, Civil Rights and Peace Activist as well as a Journalist for NE Journal Star in Lincoln, Nebraska.

- Someone to grieve for me when my heart is broken;

- Someone to carry my load when I am exhausted.

As you've probably guessed by now, I'm writing this with "tongue-in- cheek." My purpose is to point out that this is a great analogy of our spiritual relationship with God. He's the best surrogate we could find. That's because He knows our situation intimately. Since nothing is too hard for Him, He can take all of our needs and effectively meet them. He is head over heels in love with us. He cares about us.

If this seems too simplistic, I can understand. I would be the last person to try to minimize our needs as caregivers. I know personally how hard it is to ask for help; to lay down my burden; to let go and let someone else carry it for me. It's hard to believe that the answer to our needs could be so simple. But I have great news to share with you. Jesus Himself is already walking this journey with us—side by side, hand in hand. He is already our substitute, the surrogate that we so desperately need.

In Philippians 4:5-7, Paul tells us: "The Lord is near. Do not be anxious about anything, but in everything, by prayer and petition, with thanksgiving, present your request to God. And the peace of God, which transcends all understanding, will guard your hearts and minds in Christ Jesus." Praise God.

Jesus knows that as caregivers, the load of worry and anxiety is simply too heavy for us to carry alone. He knows that our heart will break beneath the weight of our sadness. He knows that our knees will buckle from the physical strain of twenty-four hour days without significant rest. He knows everything about our life.

This is the reason that He has sent us the greatest invitation we will ever receive. It is an "Invitation" to journey with Him. It is found in Matthew 11:28-30. "Come to me, all you who are weary and burdened, and I will give you rest. Take my yoke upon you and learn from me, for I am gentle and humble in heart, and you will find rest for your souls. For my yoke is easy and my burden is light."

This invitation is open to everyone who will accept it. Who would be foolish enough to turn down such a gift?

Jesus is inviting us to take whatever burden we're carrying and place it on His shoulders—a place where we can rest our head when the worries and burdens of our life try to overpower and overwhelm us.

So, instead of pulling the covers over our head and wishing that "the world would go away", let's accept this awesome invitation. Let's get out of bed and take a walk with Jesus.

Following Jesus isn't just a call to come and die. It's an invitation to live embraced by the Father, with all the privileges of being His child.

Jesus "invites us" to live with eyes wide open, always looking for evidence of His presence in the big and the small things in our lives. So, what are we waiting for: "Let's dance for Jesus; sing for Jesus; walk with Jesus; run to Jesus and live."

Difficult times may come, but He is right here through it all. Our Lord, the creator of the universe, is right at our side.

As We "Journey With Jesus" Let Us Picture This:

✝ Jesus sitting with you in the doctor's office when the doctor says the words, "It's Alzheimer's."

✝ Jesus helping you bring in the heavy groceries when you're exhausted from trying to keep up with your loved one at the store.

✝ Jesus staying beside your loved one who is lost until you can get to him.

✝ Jesus holding a mop, ready to help you clean up endless "disasters" in the bathroom.

✝ Jesus gently reminding you to eat when you're too tired and stressed to remember you haven't eaten all day.

✝ A tired caregiver who slept only three hours the night before, stretched out, resting her head on Jesus' lap while her sweetheart finally sleeps.

✝ Jesus, helping you carry heavy wet towels and blankets to the laundry room after your loved one flooded the bathroom because he couldn't shut off the water behind the overflowing commode.

✝ Jesus, wiping your tears when you sit in the car after you leave your loved one in the care of others because it is best for him.

✝ Jesus, holding the hand of an Alzheimer's sufferer because he can't remember where his room is.

✝ A lonely caregiver, whose loved one no longer recognizes her, resting her head on Jesus' shoulder.

✝ Jesus, standing beside you at the hospital all night to help you keep your loved one from climbing over the rail of his hospital bed.

✝ Jesus, standing with you at the bedside of your sweetheart, reminding you that in a few minutes He will be taking him home to Heaven to live with Him.

✝ Jesus, holding your hand as you stand at the podium during your sweetheart's funeral, sharing your story of God's faithfulness, paying tribute to your loved one.

✝ Jesus, returning home with you from the cemetery, comforting you, reminding you that your loved one is not in a cold grave but is with God, his Father, safe and well and happy.

A Special Invitation

To:	**Courageous Caregivers**
From:	**A Gracious God**
Occasion:	**A Journey with Jesus**
Where:	**Wherever You Are**
When:	**Everyday**
What Time:	**Day and Night**
Main Course:	**Comfort, Hope, Peace, Protection and Strength**
Dessert:	**Joy and Laughter**
RSVP:	**Prayer line to Heaven (Always open)**

~ Joy ~

"Joy." The very word itself lifts my spirits and makes me glad. God the Father knew that this provision would make even the most difficult part of our journey bearable.

No one has to tell us that the life of an Alzheimer's caregiver is probably one of the most difficult to endure. Not only are the days and nights long and exhausting, they are filled with disappointment and disillusionment. Dreams are shattered. The outcome is frightening. The future looks hopeless. Joy may be the last thing we expect to find, but something I desperately long to experience in the midst of my circumstance. I also long for it for James. Even in his dementia I want him to experience joy.

My Journal – May 1, 2005

I was encouraged today when I remembered that joy is a gift from God. It is a gift He has given us, one that we need only to reach out for and receive. We can choose it anytime, anywhere. In Galatians 5:22-23, Paul gives us a list of the attributes of a Christian life that he calls the fruit of the Spirit: love, joy, peace, patience, kindness, goodness, faithfulness, gentleness and self-control."

Only God could have revealed this remarkable truth to Paul—this challenge, this invitation to live our lives filled with these attributes. No wonder Paul could rejoice even while he faced constant persecution, danger, and suffering.

In Philippians 4:4 Paul tells us, "Rejoice in the Lord always. I will say it again: Rejoice." This command tells us that, even in the midst of our hardships, we can choose to rejoice. Jesus has promised to be the same—yesterday, today, and forever. That promise is a source of our joy. His life while here on earth shows us that His joy triumphs over trials.

How can we demonstrate joy in the midst of all the misery, hardships, and painful circumstances of our lives as caregivers? First, we need to understand that joy is not the same as happiness. Happiness comes and goes. Joy, on the other hand, will stay with you for the long haul. The reason? Real joy is from God. For the believer, it is like a bottomless well of water always available. Even in the darkest days, when sadness, grief, and loss may threaten to overwhelm us, God's joy is there. Like his love, it never runs out.

Second, we need to realize that, just like salvation, Joy is a free and perfect gift from God. Reach out and simply experience it. Grab onto it like a lifeline. Instead of despair, make a decision to choose joy every day. Finding "pockets of joy" each day will help us face the inevitable "why me?" moments. (Lucy)

My Journal — June 3, 2007

"Today, I need a double-serving of joy. I have found as I'm traveling this journey, that the people I meet who have the most joy don't necessarily have the easiest lives or the best of everything. They just make the best of everything that comes their way. They seem to find hope and joy even when their lives are falling apart. These people, I've discovered, have a deep faith in God. They have learned that only Jesus can give the kind of joy that comes from deep inside; from a well that never runs dry. They apparently have also found a joy that triumphs over trials. This is my goal for today and all the days ahead. I want others to see Jesus in me. I want my life to demonstrate joy, regardless of my circumstances.

Father, I know I can only do this with Your help, so I'm unapologetically asking for an extra measure of joy for today." (Lucy)

For several years, in my church, I've been teaching a Bible Study Class for older Single Adults. This past week we studied about how faith gives us our reasons to be joyful. We discussed the fact that joy does not rest in external circumstances. They know that many Sunday mornings I stand to teach after being up all night with James. For them, I am the "poster child" for finding joy. I've tried to demonstrate to them by my life that the source for joy is this truth: we are God's children, indwelled by His Spirit and joint heirs with Christ. This reality produces the joy we find in our lives. Our joy remains constant and unchanged because God's love for us remains unchanged, regardless of how easy or how difficult our lives may be.

My Journal — January 8, 2010

Whew. What a week.

Today I'm taking a break from gloom and despair. The weather for the past week has been rainy, cold, and dismal. Not only were James and I homebound physically, I was homebound emotionally. I felt as if I were in a deep, winter hibernation. Now it is time to open my heart and let God's sunlight shine in on me. So, today I choose joy. I love the way Hans Christian Andersen expressed this:

"Just living is not enough," said the butterfly,

"one must have sunshine, freedom, and a little flower."

~ Hans Christian Andersen

And I say, "Amen to this." (Lucy)

As I'm looking at this journal entry several days later, I realize that my decision to choose joy that day was the best medicine I could have received. Some of you may be asking, "Can I actually find joy in the midst of my everyday, messy, drudgery-filled life with its frustrations, disappointments and exhaustion?

- When my loved one asks if we're ever going to eat again after he or she has just eaten?

- When I've changed my loved one's clothes for the third time today?

- When my loved one uses the basket of clean clothes sitting in our bedroom because he can't find the bathroom?

- When I feel that my world is falling apart and myself along with it?

- When my loved one's questions have no end, and my questions have no answers?

My response to all of these questions is an emphatic, "Yes, you can." I can say this because they are my questions, too. I'm learning, however, that joy is not dependent on circumstances or people. It doesn't come from "hanging in there" or from "keeping a stiff upper lip." Joy doesn't even come from overcoming all the obstacles on our journey with Alzheimer's. Joy is a choice that I make as I change James' Depends; as I wash soiled sheets every day; as I mop up endless puddles; as I reassure James several times each night that we are safe.

Mother Teresa once wrote, "Joy is prayer. Joy is strength. Joy is love. Joy is a net of love by which you can catch souls."[25] I want people to see in me the very heartbeat of my joy. I want the people I encounter at the grocery store, the drugstore, the bank, the nail salon, the beauty shop, restaurants, or wherever I am, to see God's joy in me. In my countenance, my actions, my responses. I want my joy to be so contagious that others will wonder about its source and hunger for what I have found. I want to be able to respond with these words to those who wish to know my secret, "I am blessed by Jesus, who gives me supernatural health, strength, and energy to take care of my husband who has Alzheimer's. Even though my life is far from perfect, I have a Heavenly Father, who is perfect, and He gives me joy every day." The joy of the Lord is my strength (Nehemiah 8:16).

One thing that has always brought me joy is serving Jesus wherever I am needed. After James and I married, our greatest joy, other than being together, was serving, side-by-side, in our local church. Although I didn't end up going to Africa as a missionary nurse, something I had always dreamed of, I loved serving God at the side of this wonderful man He had placed in my life. I soon learned that the result of all ministry is the same—a deep sense of joy. I believe that my joy, even now, is the result of my surrender and obedience to God's calling to care for James.

As James' Alzheimer's has progressed, my ability to be involved in ministry has decreased. With God's help, I have come to accept that my most important ministry for now is caring for James and his needs. Being a full-time caregiver is not easy, but I am learning that, even through this, I can find joy. I believe that before James and I were born, God knew that someday James would have Alzheimer's. He also knew that this godly

25   *Southern Lady,* March / April 2010, p. 112.

man with the great heart would need someone to love him and to take care of him—Me.

In John 15:11, Jesus tells me that, if I am obedient to His teachings, His joy will be in me, and my joy will be complete. In John 17:13, Jesus prays for me that I will experience His joy. With His joy in my heart, I will love James and I will care for him and serve him with all my strength and energy- and joy. We find something to laugh about and to rejoice in every day. Nothing can rob us of the joy of just being together. For this blessing, I am tremendously grateful.

"Father, may you always find me on the way, not in the way, of those searching for joy in their lives, a joy that you have already given. Thank You, Father, for Your wonderful gift of joy." Amen.

My Journal — February 26, 2012

"I'm up very early. I'm editing and "polishing" the book I've been writing for four years. Later this morning, I will go over to Clare Bridge, the memory care facility, thirty seconds away, where James now lives. After almost five months there, James seems happy, loving all the attention he gets. Everyone there loves him, and he receives wonderful care. I don't worry about him, but I still miss him so much.

I'm just finishing the chapter about joy. There's a bird in a tree outside my study window. I'm listening to his beautiful song. I can't see the bird, but I can hear him. His song is sweet and joyful as he greets the morning and the sun coming up over the eastern horizon. I wonder what his song is all about. I wonder if he's singing praises to the Creator. Maybe he's praising God for another day, for life and breath, for strength to fly. Maybe he's thanking God for the food He is providing—the seeds, the bugs, whatever birds eat. Maybe he's thanking God for fellow bird friends. Only my friend, the bird, knows the answers, but I do know that he has joy that he can't contain but which he must share with all within earshot. I will take my cue from him today and "sing" with joy in my heart." (Lucy)

"You will go out in joy and be led

forth in peace; the mountains

and the hills will burst into

song before you, and all the trees of

the field will clap their hands."

~ Isaiah 55:12

~ Knowledge ~

I believe that God has given us knowledge of Himself as one of our essential provisions as we travel our journey with Alzheimer's disease. He knows that the better we know Him, the more confidently and faithfully we will follow Him. Contrary to what many so-called "self-made" individuals believe, God knows that without our knowledge of Him and His attributes, we will never be the successful travelers he has designed us to be.

I suspect that it is the cynicism of many in our present-day world which inspired Max Lucado, in his book, *In the Grip of Grace*, to include this observation:

What a Mess

"The loss of mystery has led to the loss of majesty.
The more we know, the less we believe.
No wonder there is no wonder.
We think we've figured it all out.
Strange, don't you think?
Knowledge of the workings shouldn't negate wonder.
Knowledge should stir wonder.

Who has more reason to worship than the astronomer
who has seen the stars?
Than the surgeon who has held a heart?
Than the oceanographer who has pondered the depths?"[26]

My Journal — October 29, 2009

I'm at my Bethel at sunrise. James is finally asleep after a very restless night. He is afraid of the darkness, even though I leave a night light on in our bedroom. As I sit by a large window facing east, I am watching this new day dawn with all its beauty and promise. At the moment, I am not thinking about the unknown challenges of the day. I'm not thinking about all the things I need to accomplish today. What I am thinking about is that the Lord is in His Holy Temple, watching me as I watch the sunrise. I have no doubt that He will be watching me all day long. Knowing this gives me a whole new perspective on my circumstances.

Thank You, Father, for giving me the gift of beauty and an awareness of Your presence with me today.

After watching the sunrise and thanking God for such beauty, I opened my Bible to Psalm 139, one of my favorite psalms. After reading it in its entirety, I went back and listed the truths I found there: These are things I can know about God:

✝ *He has searched me, and He knows me.*

✝ *He knows when I sit down and when I stand up.*

---

26   *In the Grip of Grace,* 1996, Max Lucado; Thomas Nelson Inc., (3 books in 1 volume), 2009.

✝ *He knows when I go out and when I lie down.*

✝ *He knows my thoughts; He is familiar with all my ways.*

✝ *He knows every word I will speak before I say it.*

✝ *He has laid His hand on me.*

✝ *I cannot go anywhere that His hand will not guide and hold me.*

✝ *Even my darkest nights are not dark to Him; He will make them shine like the day.*

✝ *He created me; He knit me together in my mother's womb. I am fearfully and wonderfully made from conception and His eyes saw my every cell as it was formed.*

✝ *All my days were written in His journal before my first day and until my last. Because of Him, my life matters.*

✝ *I am always in His thoughts, on His mind.*

✝ *When I awake each day, I am with God.*

✝ *He searches my heart and knows when I am anxious or stressed. He knows all the secret, empty places in my heart.*

✝ *He points out my offensive thoughts and actions and leads me in His way forever.*

As I read over my 'paraphrase' of this beautiful Psalm 139, I sense that my heavenly Father is telling me, personally, that I'm special to Him, that He is always nearby, involved in everything I do and everything that concerns me. He is telling me that today He will be walking with me as I face the challenges of living each moment consumed with the dementia of James' Alzheimer's. (Lucy)

☙❧

Every time I open God's Word, especially to the *Psalms,* I hear His voice. He makes me promises; tells me truths; gives me the answers He knows I need, just when I need them. He assures me that nothing is too hard for Him; that I will never face anything He has not faced; that I will never go anywhere that He has not already been. As David so transparently stated in *Psalm 139:6,* "Such knowledge is too wonderful for me, too lofty for me to attain." I pray that you, too, may hear, if you haven't already, that God is eagerly waiting to speak to you in your season of need.

In the book of *Job,* we hear Job say, in the midst of his grief, torment, and suffering: "I know that my Redeemer lives and that in the end he will stand upon the earth" (Job 19:25). If Job can make this statement of faith as he endured every kind of loss imaginable, I, too, can say in the midst of my loss: "Father, I know that you live in my heart and my everyday life. These are things you have personally revealed to me:

✝ *I am not alone, even when I am lonely.*

✝ *Your peace is available to me when I am anxious.*

✝ *When I need wisdom, all I have to do is ask You.*

✝ *When my heart is broken, You understand my grief.*

✝ *When I am afraid, You are my refuge.*

✝ *When I am weak, You are my strength.*

✝ *When I am lost, You are my Shepherd.*

✝ *When I am in a dark place, You are my Light.*

✝ *When I am in a storm, You are my anchor and safe harbor.*

✝ *When I am lonely, You are my best Friend.*

✝ *When this life is over, You will be waiting for me at Heaven's gate.*

These are indispensable truths that God the Father wants us to know. Otherwise, where else can we go to find comfort when our world falls apart, when the unthinkable happens? Where else can we turn when the diagnosis: "It's Alzheimer's," knocks us off our feet and changes our future forever?

Our heavenly Father knows that caregiving can be very stressful. He knows that we have unlimited reasons to be anxious and fearful. He knows that there will be times as we care for our loved one when "storms will rage" and we will wonder if He is "asleep at the helm." Those are the times when we are tempted to doubt if He is present in our difficult, drudgery-filled days.

It has been at those times during my journey that I have realized that God is not only all that I have; He is all that I need, and He is more than enough.

With that realization has come the ability to view even the worst, most devastating situation as my "gateway" to a new, more intimate relationship with Him.

In the months following James' diagnosis, I had no place to go, no one to turn to except my heavenly Father. As I desperately clung to Him, it was as if He began to peel away the layers of my previous perception of Him and to reveal deeper things about Himself that He wanted me to know.

I began to keep a daily spiritual growth journal, one that would track my progress as I grew in my deeply personal knowledge of God. This book is, in part, the culmination of that growth tracking, that search for a relationship deeper than any I had ever experienced. I called it my "experiential pursuit."

During my pursuit, I learned to trust God, even when everything seemed to be "falling apart", and I couldn't see or hear Him; when nothing made sense. When He asked me to sell my "miracle house", something which seemed at the time to be illogical and unreasonable, I still trusted Him. After all, I had trusted Him to lead me to this "perfect house" on Rainbow Bend.

If I've told this story before, please bear with me. In the spring of 1999, testing showed that James had suffered, in recent months, a left frontal lobe stroke. When his neurologist suggested that we move out of our large two-story house, we began looking for a one-story house in communities with new homes. There was a new community adjacent to the grounds of a wonderful, fast-growing church. As we turned into the community, we stopped at the first cross street, and I prayed: "Lord, please show us a four-bedroom house with a detached garage, facing north on a street where there are no more vacant lots on which to build. We turned right on that street, Rainbow Bend (I loved the name.), and within the first block we found our "perfect house." We bought it the next day.

It is perfectly natural, as believers, to want to know God's will for our lives. Instead of always trying to find His will, however, we must first find God Himself. One of my favorite scriptures is Psalm 46:10: "Be still, and know that I am God." We may not have a literal "burning bush" experience, as Moses did, but we have something infinitely better. We have God Himself living within us in the person of the Holy Spirit. We also have the complete Word of God contained in the sixty-six books of the Bible, something the Old Testament patriarchs did not have.

Just knowing that God is unshakable, unchanging, all knowing, all powerful, and that He will never leave us or forsake us, is enough to enable us to walk with complete confidence into the future, no matter how dark or uncertain the path we travel.

~ Laughter ~

Below is a replica of a poster that hung on the Medication Room door at Clare Bridge, The Hampton at Pearland, where James lived from October 1, 2011 to September 17, 2012

"Wanted"

JAMES DISHONGH

"CRIME"

STEALING HEARTS

"REWARD"

One undisturbed hour with
Mr. James, as he asks
over and over and over:
"Have you always been that
pretty? - or - that wonderful?"

~ Living Hilariously in a Dark Time ~

I read somewhere, "Silence is golden, but laughter is priceless." I totally agree. Also, I firmly believe that a day is incomplete without laughter.

I'm so glad that God packed this provision for our journey. He knew that we would need all the laughter He would graciously provide. Our responsibility is to unpack this provision daily, regardless of our circumstances. None of us need a doctor to tell us that laughter and a happy heart help us to feel better. God's Word tell us:

"A cheerful heart is good medicine, but a crushed
spirit dries up the bones"
(Proverbs 17:22).

Although the ability to laugh does not depend on what is happening in our lives, sometimes it's difficult to find a reason to laugh when we're in a sad, dark place. At times, it may even feel inappropriate. When our loved one suffers from Alzheimer's disease, our lives are drastically changing and steadily unraveling.

As caregiver to our special one, our stress level is extremely high, making the gift of laughter even more important. Laughter has been shown to cause changes in our hormones that lower our stress level and release in our body endorphins, known as feel-good chemicals.

Laughter is not only a lot less expensive than medication, we can never overdose on it. In the precious movie, "Mary Poppins", Uncle Albert sang this reminder, "The more I laugh, the more I fill with glee and the more the glee, the more I'm a merrier me." Don't you just love it?

God has joy and laughter reserved for us as we seek Him in the midst of our despair. He knows that our hearts are raw from watching Alzheimer's ravage and steadily destroy the very essence of the person who was once our healthy, bright parent, spouse or sibling. He knows that our needs are deep, enormous, and endless. This is precisely the reason that our Father, the Great Physician, prescribes laughter.

I'm writing this chapter on July 22, 2012, my seventy-eighth birthday and the thirteenth anniversary of James' diagnosis. I went to Clare Bridge this morning to have breakfast with James and to see the other dear people there. They are now like a part of our "family." One sweet lady, Martha, had on her apron. I call her the "Homemaker of the Year." She is in a wheelchair, but she "plans meals for her large family." She told me she "needed to get home because everyone was coming to her house for dinner tonight."

As I watched these precious few, each with their own personalities, I realized that a special part of each one is still intact, despite their dementia. I watched as James reached over and took his "neighbor's" bacon. I said, "Honey, don't take Tim's food." James said, "He doesn't want it. I'm starved. You know I haven't eaten for three days." Then he got so tickled, he almost choked on Tim's bacon. The care associates and I laughed, too.

Sometimes, we just have to laugh. Even when our life changes and goes in a direction we would have never chosen, if we try, we can still find joy and humor.

As I looked in the mirror this morning at my seventy-eight-year old face, I was reminded that God has a sense of humor. Even though I feel thirty-eight, physically and mentally, I could use a facelift. Then I smiled at my reflection as God reminded me that a smile is better than Botox or a facelift and a lot less painful and expensive.

Today, I will look for reasons to smile and to laugh because I believe that God created me for laughter. I'm suddenly reminded of a story in Genesis 21 about Sarah, the wife of Abraham. She was much older than I am today when she became pregnant with Isaac. I'm wondering which was worse—her "morning sickness" or her rheumatism.

I'm sharing part of her story, told in today's language: "Push, Sarah," the midwife said. Sarah pushed and in an instant, the child entered the world. "It's a boy, Sarah," one of the women cried. "It's a boy. And he looks just like you: wrinkled and toothless." Sarah heard the baby's first cry and her weary, old body shook with laughter. Sometimes you just have to laugh. Life takes off in an unexpected, even unbelievable direction, but you just have to laugh [27]

Sarah's life certainly did not turn out as she had planned. I'm very sure of that. But she found a reason to laugh. I'm also sure that she found much joy in Isaac, that baby boy born in her old age, a baby whose name means "he laughs."

Even though life, as James and I knew it, has been steadily changing and unraveling for the past thirteen years, he and I have laughed often. Even now, laughter bubbles up without warning, and we are wonderfully uplifted and blessed.

Job 8:21 tells us, "He (God) will yet fill your mouth with laughter and your lips with shouts of joy." I've always believed that there should be a lot of laughter in a home, even one where dementia dwells. Nothing can relieve the inevitable tension that comes from twenty-four hours of caregiving more than a good laugh. I can think of times when I was ready

---

27   *Risk the Journey*, by Bill J. Leonard, 101, (Woman's Missionary Union, Birmingham, AL, 1995).

to "strangle" James that he would say something hilarious, and we would have a good laugh.

Incidentally, did you know that laughter is good exercise? I have read that it is like jogging on the inside. I much prefer that to jogging on the outside, especially in Houston's humidity. (A little humor.)

Let's take time out here for a little "inside jog." I want to share with you a story that never fails to make me laugh, even though I have read and shared it many times.

Luci Swindoll, one of the Women of Faith speakers, tells the story. She and Marilyn Meberg, another of the Women of Faith speakers, were in Luci's kitchen one Christmas. Luci asked Marilyn for her favorite recipe. "Without the slightest hesitation, Marilyn said, "Okay, write this down"—and Luci did.

Marilyn's Favorite Recipe for Smooth and Satiny Brown Gravy

4 cups of flour
1 cup fruit cocktail (with liquid)
1 Tablespoon white pepper
1 teaspoon nutmeg
3 Tablespoons of salt
1 cup of arrowroot
2 teaspoons of cinnamon
1 cup of raisins

Take a 5-pound mallet, place in the palm of your right hand. Methodically coerce lumps into satiny submission. Allow one hour for smooth and satiny effect. May be made ahead of time and stored until the return of Christ. Serve in silver, which enhances flavor. Serve 23 guests, give or take 12. (Aunt Rebecca commented after four bites: "Something's amiss, but…"—after which she slipped quietly into a coma.)[28]

---

28   *Boundless Love*, p. 167, Zondervan Publishing House, Grand Rapids, Michigan, 2001.

Like Luci, I "love, love, love that outlandish recipe." I, too may "make that gravy someday and not only slip into a coma, but die a happy woman."[29]

I sincerely hope that this gave you a laugh and a break from despair. I read it to my sister recently on the phone when she was having a "blah" day. She is an excellent cook, and I knew she would appreciate it. By the time I finished reading it, we were both laughing hysterically.

"Thank you, Luci and Marilyn, for sharing your wonderful gifts of humor with others."

As my priorities have gradually changed during the past thirteen years, I've learned to laugh at myself more easily and to not be so hard on myself. As a Christian woman, I want to be exceptional where God is concerned, but I have learned that there are boundaries I don't need to cross. He already has those things covered. I've discovered this truth during the countless hours I've spent at His feet the last thirteen years.

I've learned to "let go" and let God. I'm surrendering to Him the burdens which I still think, at times, I must carry.

More and more I'm learning to experience the joy of the Lord and to look for the humor in others and myself. My precious James has taught me this—this man who, even after years of the ravages of Alzheimer's, can laugh at himself and others, creating a sense of wonder and joy in his presence.

James has always had a dry sense of humor. It is one of the qualities that has endeared him to me and our children, and to others, for as long as I have known him. Even now, his friends will often ask, "Does James still have his wonderful sense of humor?" As an answer, I will share with them one of his latest "hilarities."

---

29   Ibid.

By the year 2004, James had begun to lose some of his usual inhibitions. Although he had always been a friendly, charming man with a dry sense of humor, he was also rather quiet, reserved, and thoughtful. He would have done nothing to call attention to himself. Now, it was as if the "real" James began to evolve. In contrast to many Alzheimer's sufferers, however, he was never hateful, crude, or vulgar. He just became more and more childlike and "innocent" in his advancing dementia.

The rest of this chapter consists of laughter-inducing journal entries which track the evolution of James' noteworthy sense of humor. I call it: "James Dishongh's Strategy for Living Hilariously in a Dark Time."

July 18, 2004: "Starting about three months ago, when we go to a restaurant, James always asks our waitress, "Have you always been that pretty?" Sometimes he will say, "Do I have to pay extra since you're so beautiful?" Today, while at a restaurant having breakfast with friends from our church, James looked intently at the not especially attractive waitress approaching our table. We all held our breath until James asked her, "Have you always had that beautiful smile?" We almost fell out of our chairs with relief and laughter. The waitress looked very pleased—so did James."

March 3, 2006: "This morning, while James was occupied with reading the newspaper, I went to take a shower and wash my hair. When I returned to the kitchen in about twenty-five minutes, James was eating a banana. I looked over at the fruit basket and realized that, where there had been four or five bananas, now there were none. I said, "James, what happened to the rest of the bananas?" James looked up innocently and said, "I don't know." I looked in the kitchen trashcan and saw five banana peelings. I said, "James, you ate all the bananas this morning. Eating that many bananas is not good for you." Proclaiming his innocence, James got up to look in the trashcan. He said "I didn't eat those. Someone must have come in while I wasn't looking. They ate all of our bananas." He went to check the back door and came back to report, "They're gone. We'll never find them." By now, I was trying to hide my amusement. It was frustrating but so funny. I said, "Maybe the person who came in and ate all our bananas will have a stomach ache." James said, "I hope so." After today, I will store the bananas in our guest bedroom across the hall."

June 1, 2007: "Today, the doorbell rang and before I could get to the door, James had already opened it. He was talking to a woman who, by the time I got there, was almost doubled over with laughter. She explained that she was with the cable company and had come to bury the phone line at the side of our house. When she told James that she had come to bury the line, he had said to her, "I didn't know it was dead." Then we all had a good laugh."

May 2, 2008: "We have an appointment today with James' urologist. I was helping James dry off after his shower when he looked at me and asked, "Am I your little boy?" I said, "No, you're my husband." James replied, "Boy, am I lucky." Later, at the doctor's office, we had to wait longer than usual. When the doctor finally came into the examining room, James said, "You must have had to walk a long way to get here. You need to get a car." Then he said, "I'm sure glad I'm not bald like you." The doctor and I just shook our head and smiled."

September 14, 2009: "This morning I was encouraging James to finish dressing so that we could walk to the mailbox before the mailman comes. After I had become slightly annoyed with him, he said, "You can't expect too much from me. I have Alzheimer's, you know." The new word for the day is "Is-was." James woke up asking, "Am I an 'Is was?'" On the way to the mailbox down the block from our home, we talked about his new word. (Frequently a new word "pops up," and I tease him about rewriting the English language.) I asked James, "What language is 'Is-was'?" James said, "Alzheimer's of course." Then he got so tickled, he got out of breath and had to hold on to me. He said, "If I ever get home, I'm never leaving again." I'm so glad God has provided laughter for us.

September 15, 2009: "James enjoys going to the grocery store with me, but lately, he gets tired after a few minutes. Today I left him home with our oldest son. I was gone about an hour, and when I returned, James said, "I'm leaving. I'm packed and ready to go." When I asked our son what was wrong, he said, "Dad was upset that you were gone. He said," If she's not back in a few minutes, I'm going to be madder than a wet hen." Then he went to your room and "packed." (He had stuffed three or four handkerchiefs into his pockets.) Then he came back and sat down to wait for you." When I told James that I was sorry he was leaving because I had bought his favorite ice cream, he said, "I guess I'll stay." I hugged him, and we both laughed."

October 5, 2009: "Today I have an appointment with my Ophthalmologist. This means that I must not only get myself ready, I must also get James showered, shaved, and dressed. As I was shaving James, he said, "I've never been shaved by a beautiful woman. Do I know you?" When I said, "Yes", he said, "What's your name?" I don't know where it came from, but I said, "Sassafras Tea." James started laughing and couldn't stop. He finally sat down on the floor, shaving cream and all. I laughed, too, and it felt so good. I made a decision then and there to keep things light and happy for as long as possible. Later, at the Eye Clinic, James was his usual charming self. Within minutes of arriving, despite my warning, James had asked everyone in the waiting room their name, how long they had been there, and if they were okay. By the time we were ready to leave the clinic, he had told every nurse he saw that she was "beautiful and could stop taking her beauty pills." In the background, unknown to me, the young clinic manager had been observing James. As we checked out at the desk, the manager came over, shook James' hand and introduced himself. James asked him, "Are you real?" Recovering quickly, the young man said, "Yes, I'm real." Then James said "No, you're too wonderful to be real." James said, "You sure are dressed up. Have you always been that…(James hesitated; I knew his mind was trying to find an appropriate word—somehow he knew "pretty" was not it.) Then he finished: "Have you always been that remarkable?" We all laughed, and the desk clerk applauded. I could tell that the young manager was moved. He said to James, "You're the one that's remarkable." Then he winked at me and said, "You're very blessed." Although I was exhausted by the time I drove home through five- o'clock traffic, fed James, and got him ready for bed, (all this with "dilated eyes"), I could say to James, "This has been a wonderful day, one filled with laughter and joy." And he said, "Amen."

August 1, 2010: "James had an appointment with his Urologist today. The waiting room is not very large, and by the time we arrived, it was almost filled. James is delighted when he is with people and he wastes no time getting acquainted. It doesn't take long for him to know everything about them they are willing to share. In the midst of this getting "acquainted period," one of the nurses walked through and said, "Hello, Mr. Dishongh." James looked around and said, "Everyone knows me; I'm so popular." A nicely dressed man sitting across the room from us said, "Mrs. Dishongh, you should have your own "reality TV show." It would win an Emmy." Everyone laughed, even James, although he didn't quite get the joke. As I sat there, I thought about the laughter and joy that James creates everywhere he goes. It's at times like this I can honestly say, "Thank You, God, for Alzheimer's."

September 5, 2010: "Because today is James' eighty-fourth birthday, I picked him up early from Clare Bridge so that he could have dinner with me next door in our building's dining room. (He had already had a party at Clare Bridge.) We had chocolate chip cookies for dessert. James ate his two cookies and then looked longingly at mine. James said, "I sure would like some more cookies." I said, "If you are good, you can have mine." After thinking for a moment, James said, "How good do I have to be?" Everyone within earshot laughed hysterically. Needless to say, James got my cookies." Later that day, I walked over to Clare Bridge to check on James' medications. While I was sitting on a love seat with him, the male nurse walked by, and James asked, "Who are you?" The nurse said, "I'm Lisa." James said, "That's a girl's name and besides, you're not all that pretty." At this we all laughed, including James, who sometimes laughs so hard, he loses his breath."

December 3, 2011: "One of the Care Associates at Clare Bridge where James now lives full time, called for a medication refill. When I asked her about James, she laughed and told me what he had said to a group who had come that day to sing for the residents there. One of them had walked up to James and said, "Hello, James." James said, "How do you know me?" As he looked around at the group, he said, "Everyone knows me. I must be somebody very important." Of course, they loved it, and they laughed appreciatively, she reported."

June 4, 2012: "Earlier, I was at Clare Bridge having lunch with James. One of my favorite Care Associates came over to the table to share something James had said the night before. These are her words: "I was walking James down the hall to his room to get him ready for bed. When I told him that he was walking like a little old man, he laughed and said, 'well, I am an 18-year-old Senior Citizen.'" The same women shared another recent incident involving James. She said that "one day, James was convinced that I had "front gated" him and "cheated him out of 20%." No one could figure out what he meant by "front gated" until she noticed that *Frontgate* was the name of the magazine he was reading. They thought that was hysterical.

August 27, 2012: "The Care Associate assigned to care for James today could "scarcely wait" for me to arrive so that she could share about him. As she was giving him his morning shower, he said to her, "You're too beautiful to be naked." While she was still laughing about that remark, James asked her name. She said, "What does my name tag say?" Then James said, "I didn't know it could talk?"

These are only a few of the many things I could have shared with you. It was these funny little things along our path that helped me get through each day. They are things I will remember forever. Write down your funny stories and good memories from your own journey. I think you will be surprised when you realize that this provision of laughter was there all the time.

P.S. James always knows that our sons and grandsons are someone special that he should know, but he doesn't always remember their names or their relationship to him. Our middle son, who is the most like his Dad, teases him and makes him laugh. When James asks him who he is, he says, "I'm your son." And James says, "you're not shining." It's a standing joke between them. When our grandson, Adam, tells James his name, James asks, "Where's Eve."

James' Frequent Questions and Obsessions

- "Do we live here are just stay here?"

- "Have you figured out who I am? I'm not Turkey Izgit."

- "Do we get anything to eat today? 'Yes' or 'No?'"

- "Do I stay here until something happens? Or what?"

- "Am I a lost cause? I hate to be a lost cause, but I don't know what that is."

- "Do you remember that I'm a nothing and a nobody? What is a 'nobody' anyway?"

- "Do I get anything to eat before I starve to death? You know I haven't eaten for three days?"

- "Am I a legal citizen? Am I? Are you sure?"

- "Do we have any lights? Why is it so dark?" (2:00 a.m.)

- "You haven't cut off my food supply have you? I guess I'll just starve to death. I hate to die this young." (83 years of age)

- "Am I retired? I'm not old enough to retire. Don't tell me how old I am; I don't want to know. Did I work at Shell? (40 years) Am I the President? Do I work today? I better get dressed."

I have to add one more story about my precious James. Several days after I moved James to Clare Bridge, I received a phone call at 8:30 P.M. from one of the Care Associates there. She told me that James refused to go to bed without first talking to his wife. She said to him, "I don't know your wife or her phone number." James said, "I can't remember her name, but her number is (our phone number, one we have had for years)."

~ Light ~

When God created the earth, He knew that His creation would need light, and He took care of that need on the first day. "And God said, 'Let there be light', and there was light" (Genesis 1:3). With those words, God gave us the sun, the moon and the stars (Genesis 1:16).

We all know that light is essential for life in both the animal and the plant kingdom. Light or the lack thereof affects our moods. In winter, shorter days can create a "Seasonal Affective Disorder," a common depression caused by less exposure to natural sunlight. We've all experienced this to some extent when nature gives us a series of cloudy, gloomy days without sunshine. When the sun finally comes out again, our mood automatically lifts.

While light represents joy and safety, darkness somehow represents danger. I remember a period in my childhood when I was terrified of the dark. It was probably a two-fold problem. First, it was during the era of the Wolfman and Werewolf movies. Second, we had moved to a new home in a new city. Even after all these years, I can remember dreading the time each night when my mother tucked me into bed, said my prayers with me, kissed me goodnight and turned out the light. She always said, "Don't be afraid. Remember, Daddy and I are right across the hall."

Now, seventy years later, I live with my husband, my "little man" who suffers from Alzheimer's disease, and who dreads the inevitable darkness of night. Every night, at bedtime, he starts asking, "Do you think we're safe? Are you sure? How do you know?" Most nights, he wakes me at 2:00 or 3:00 A.M. with the same questions.

When this first occurred in 2004, I recognized it as the onset of sundowning; also referred to as Sundown Syndrome. As a nurse, I had witnessed this symptom, (it isn't a 'disease'), in elderly patients who had come from surgery or who suffered from senility or dementia.

Sundowning, which affects 20% of all Alzheimer's patients, is a psychological phenomenon associated with restlessness and confusion. It generally occurs when the sun goes down and sometimes through the night. (James' usually occurred during the night.) You can see that this syndrome prevents people with dementia from sleeping well. It also makes them more likely to get up and wander around during the night.

Due to the stress that it puts on caregivers, you can see why sundowning is a common cause of caregiver burnout. (How true.)

The side effects are numerous and varied. Every sufferer of sundowning is different, with needs unique to their situation. Therefore, there is not just one simple approach or treatment. According to doctors at John Hopkins University School of Medicine, there is not even a clear definition of what "Sundown Syndrome" means. It is simply a phrase that covers a multitude of symptoms.

Because of this conclusion, I believe that, as caregivers, we must be sensitive to our loved one's symptoms and we must be flexible and willing to adapt. Some of the side effects are:

- Confusion

- Delirium

- Agitation and outbursts, anger

- Anxiety

- Restlessness

- Hallucinations

- Paranoia (Thankfully, James was never angry or paranoid.)

- Depression, crying, sadness

- Pacing, wandering, shadowing

Possible Causes of Sundowning

- All medical professionals agree that it has something to do with the onset of darkness.

- Some believe that the syndrome is an accumulation of all the sensory stimulation from the day that begins to overwhelm and cause stress.

- Others speculate that it can be caused by hormonal imbalances that occur at night.

- Some believe that the onset of symptoms at night is simply due to fatigue.

- Others believe that it has to do with anxiety caused by the inability to see well in the dark and the shadows that appear at night in certain parts of the room.

Practical Advice to Help Caregivers Handle Symptoms and Lessen the Effects:

- Always use a calm, soothing approach.

- Because some research suggests that symptoms may be related to changes to the brain's circadian pacemaker, a cluster of nerve cells that keep the body on a 24-hour clock, it makes sense that a consistent, regular routine is crucial. It alleviates anxiety and makes them feel safe.

- Plan activities during the day, such as light exercise and walking. At Clare Bridge, the Memory Care facility at the Brookdale Community where James lived for two years, the residents played balloon volleyball inside. After lunch, they walked outside around the garden, where they could plant flowers or fill the bird feeders.

- Discourage long daytime naps. (Lots of luck.)

- Encourage any hobby that gets your loved one up and moving. I took James with me to the beauty shop, nail salon, the mall.

- Plan a healthy diet; make sure your loved one eats properly. Left to himself, James would have lived on Snickers, chocolate chip cookies, ice cream, and bananas.

- Limit caffeine and sugar to morning hours.

- Have regular medical checkups. Because sundowning seems to be more pronounced with pain, severe constipation, certain medications, and infection, have the doctors check for infection, especially Urinary Tract Infections. Also, have them review prescription medications frequently; check for signs of constipation to avoid fecal impactions.

- Late afternoon, close drapes so that your loved one can't see the sky change from light to dark. Turn on inside lights at dusk to keep the environment light and calm.

- Provide a peaceful setting. Try to prevent or reduce excessive noise during sunset.

One of the proven, most necessary treatments for sundowning is light therapy. Exposure to bright lights, like daylight, may reduce some symptoms, especially when used in combination with exercise, like walking.

Every day, for ten years, until we moved from our home on Rainbow Bend to the Hampton, James and I walked down the block to our mailbox. Many days, we walked around the block. On cloudy, gloomy days, we often went to one of the malls or Wal-Mart to walk. (James loved people.) On rainy days, I turned on all the lights in the house, and we played dominoes or read. James loved the daily newspaper and would read it over and over all day. Sometimes, to keep James moving, I put in a favorite CD, and we danced. (Neither of us were good dancers, but we laughed at our efforts, and we had fun.)

At night, I turned on our bathroom light and a night light in our bedroom. If James was unusually restless or anxious or got out of bed, looking for "something", (once, it was a 'clock'), we would sit in our side-by- side recliners in our bedroom (and sometimes sleep there). I would talk to him, reminding him how God was watching over us all the time, especially at night. Sometimes I sang softly to him-he loved "Amazing Grace." Even when I was exhausted and sleep deprived, I tried to be "cool, calm and collected." The only way I could do this was to constantly remind myself:

When James is fearful at dusk, following me around the house in the evening (shadowing me); when he asks the same questions over and over again during the night, he is not purposely trying to stress or aggravate me. This is simply something he can't help.

To reassure James and to alleviate his feeling of never being safe, I had a security system installed in our Rainbow Bend house. It verbally told me, day or night, if an outside door was opened. At night, I always kept James with me in our bedroom. We slept together in our king-sized Tempur-Pedic bed. (It was two twins fitted together in a king-size, four poster bed frame.) I know that some caregivers choose to sleep in a separate room, especially if the patient is a parent or sibling. This is certainly understandable-baby monitor's work well in this case. Recently, I read a statement on Google, "The only difference between Pediatrics and Geriatrics is 'body mass'."

Each morning, after a troubled night, I went straight to my "Bethel", my blue chair in the Living Room where I met God each morning. Here He pointed out scriptures in His Word. One of my favorites: "The Lord is my light and my salvation; whom shall I fear? The Lord is the stronghold of my life—of whom shall I be afraid?" (Psalm 27:1)

As I'm writing this, I'm reminded of a perfect example of how God provides light where we need it the most: "In October of 2002,

James and I took a chartered bus tour up the East Coast with about fifty friends from our previous church. We were scheduled to spend the first night at a Holiday Inn in Meridian, Mississippi. Before checking in, we stopped at a special restaurant for dinner. We could see the lights of our motel in the distance.

While we were having dinner, a thunderstorm with heavy rain, wind, and lightning struck the area. Thankfully, by the time we finished dinner and boarded the bus, the storm had passed. As we headed in the direction of our motel, it was apparent that something was different. There were no lights. When we reached the now dark Holiday Inn, we were informed that, because of the storm, there had been a "black out" in that block and several other motels and businesses were affected. We were assured that Light Company trucks were on the way to fix the problem.

James was exhausted and, although some chose to remain on the bus, he and I decided, along with several others, to try to find our rooms. With the help of these friends and with borrowed flashlights, James and I made our way up the outdoor stairway to our second-floor room. When I unlocked the door, the room was "entirely black." I felt my way carefully across the room and opened the drapery. The room was instantly flooded with light.

Much to my amazement and delight, the windows looked out on a Shell Service Station with its large, bright red and yellow "Pectin" sign. This was a familiar "friend" from the forty years James was employed by Shell Oil Company. The company symbol, the Pectin, is displayed throughout our home on plaques, books, and other decorative objects.

I will always be convinced that only God could have orchestrated something so perfect and so amazing to demonstrate His presence with us that night. It was a night when I was feeling "fragile" and desperately needed that "sign" from the Lord.

The day in 1999 when the doctor said the words, "It's Alzheimer's," I was caught in the grip of fear. The darkness that seemed to surround me at that moment reminded me of a bright, sunny day suddenly made dark by a black cloud covering the sun. As the "dark clouds" of Alzheimer's began to move over our lives, they threatened to block out the light and peace in our safe, predictable world.

James and I knew we needed God to shine His light on our path as we began this strange, new journey into the dark unknowns of Alzheimer's disease. We turned to Jesus, the Light of the world, and asked Him to supply the light we would need—and He did.

Even in our darkest nights, we knew we were being led by an unseen hand. We also knew that when we trusted Him, we didn't need to see the whole path, just the part we would be traveling each day.

I love, love, love this quote by Helen Keller, deaf and blind from birth, but a powerful, constant inspiration, even in death: "Dark as my path may seem to others, I carry a magic light in my heart. Faith, the spiritually strong search light, illumines the way and, although sinister doubts lurk in the shadow, I walk unafraid."

When "darkness" comes, (and it will), if we turn to God for guidance, He will walk with us through our darkness, and we will come out stronger and victorious on the other side. I realized that I have developed more during this "darkness" of Alzheimer's than at any other time in my life. If we will "hang on" and wait for morning, joy will come. This is a promise found in Psalm 30:5 AMP, "Weeping may endure for a night, but joy comes in the morning."

My Journal — September 8, 2009

"In the early stages of James' illness, he still functioned well during the day with a little help from me. As time passed, there were things that he began to have difficulty accomplishing; things that required logic and reasoning. He could no longer pay bills, balance the checkbook, prepare our tax return, or use his camera. In 2004, at his doctor's request, he no longer drove, something that he accepted with no complaint.

To the casual observer, James was entirely normal. The nights were a different story. As soon as it began to get dark, James became anxious and restless because of Sundown Syndrome. During the long, troubled nights I grieved. I longed for the nights before Alzheimer's when I could crawl into bed beside James and feel safe and contented. We slept like spoons nestled together. In those days, I could not have imagined life any other way. James was so steady, dependable, confident and strong. With him I always felt safe—he was my protector.

Now, our roles are reversed. During my sleepless nights when James is restless, even in sleep; when he moves frequently and mumbles; when he touches my arm to be sure I'm still there, my mind is wide-awake. I pray, recite familiar Bible verses, compose poetry, mentally pay bills and most of all, worry about the future. The uncertainty and unknowns of the future are becoming something to dread. I'm always grateful when the first light of the new day appears, and James settles into a peaceful sleep. If I let him, he would sleep until noon.

Here at my "Bethel" this morning, I'm praying this prayer, "Father, today as I face difficult decisions and problems, I'm asking for Your light to dispel the dimness of my logic and reasoning. You already know that I must supply for both of us what James has lost. I need for You to light my path today when my vision becomes blurred and clouded by stress and exhaustion. Thank You, Father, for being my guiding light."
(Lucy)

My Journal — October 18, 2010

"This morning in my quiet time, I read Psalm 19:1, "The heavens declare the glory of God; the skies proclaim the work of His hand." Tonight, after a Care Associate walked James over from Clare Bridge to our apartment at the Hampton, I met him at our door, and we walked across the hall and out

onto the open deck. I wanted James to see the night sky filled with stars and the beautiful Autumn moon. When James and I were engaged, in October of 1957, we loved sitting on the hood of his car at Hermann Park, looking at the stars, watching the October moon rise, talking for hours. Tonight, as we watched that same moon that we watched fifty-three years ago, I realized again how blessed we are to have found one another. As I talked to James about the stars and the moon that God has put in the sky to give light to our world and our lives, James said, "Thank You, Lord." I said, "God loves us so much he created the moon and the stars so that our nights would never be dark." James said, "Amen" and clapped his hands. It was a precious time." (Lucy)

My Journal — October 19, 2010

"During the night, awake because of James' restlessness, I thought about the words of the song which made Debbie Boone famous back in 1977—the much loved "You Light Up My Life", by Joe Brooks:

In my mind, I sang these words as a praise to God, my Father. In return, He reminded me that even though "darkness" has come into my life, my faith in Him will enable me to walk through this darkness of Alzheimer's. He promised that He will turn the "light" on as I spend time with Him in His Word. Thank You Father for this new day and the joy and energy I am experiencing this morning in spite of a serious lack of sleep. You are an awesome God." (Lucy)

Remember with me, "shadows can frighten us, but they can't hurt us. When the sun goes down, we know that it will come back in the morning. Wait for it. God doesn't need our help to do this, but He wants our faith and trust."

Above all, remember: "this, too, shall pass." Every morning at my "Bethel", I ask God for patience, endurance and strength for the day-and the night. I also thank Him for Thomas Edison.

I want to close this very long chapter with some priceless words spoken by Betsie ten Boom and recorded by her sister, Corrie ten Boom in her book, *Amazing Love*. She spoke these words in the horrible darkness of a German Concentration Camp, where she died during the Holocaust: "The most important part of our task will be to tell everyone who will listen that Jesus is the only answer to the problems that are disturbing the hearts of man and nations. We shall have the right to speak because we can tell from our experiences that his light is more powerful than the deepest darkness. How beautiful that the reality of his presence is greater than the reality of the hell about us."[30]

~ Miracles ~

Recently, while shopping, I saw this thought-provoking message on a decorative plaque: "Every day holds the possibility of a miracle." My first thought was, "Yes. I want to experience miracles. I want to see God's power in my circumstances."

I'm sure we all do. I believe in miracles because I have a Father in heaven who specializes in them. The Bible is filled with stories of His miracles. They are an integral part of the Bible. There are more than one hundred and fifty accounts scattered throughout the Old and New Testaments. These miracles cover all types of human needs: protection, intervention, deliverance, healing, provision, and transformation.

I have my own stories. You probably have yours. Think about it: every miracle starts with a problem or a need. I believe that God wants us to experience His supernatural intervention in our lives when we have a need only He can meet. Not as a "magician", but as a powerful, loving Father. The good news is that we don't need an appointment to get a miracle from God. He will see us and our need, whatever the need, wherever we are.

One thing I've learned during our thirteen-year journey with Alzheimer's: God chooses the miracle He knows we need. After James'

30   Quoted in *Women's Devotional Bible,* NIV, Copyright 1990, 1994, The Zondervan Corporation, p. 1278.

diagnosis, I prayed earnestly for miraculous healing for him. I knew that nothing was too hard for God. But God chose, instead, to give James the miracle of a sweet, gentle spirit and disposition for the entire thirteen years.

God enabled him to touch everyone he met with his God-given love and his wonderful sense of humor. His life with Alzheimer's was an example of the fact that many people with a strong faith in God do not always experience divine healing. They are, however, blessed with the power to continue to live with joy and dignity, even in the dementia of Alzheimer's.

Webster's New 20th Century Dictionary defines a miracle as "an event or effect that apparently contradicts known scientific laws and is hence thought to be due to supernatural causes especially to an act of God."

Billy Graham, in *The Gift of Miracles,* defines a miracle as "an event beyond the power of any known physical law to produce; it is a spiritual occurrence produced by the power of God, a marvel, a wonder."[31]

In that same publication, John Foster describes miracles as "the great bell of the universe, which draws man to God's sermon.[32]

My favorite is a quote from George MacDonald: "The miracles of Jesus were the ordinary works of His Father, wrought small and swift that we might take them in."[33]

In light of all this, it's interesting to think about all the things we call miracles, when they are just evidence of God's love for us. The truth is, He wants us to know that He is personally involved in everything that happens in our everyday lives.

One example of this is finding a parking place in front of the store when it's raining. I'll admit, I pray for this quite often. And, more often than not, the parking place appears, just as I need it. Another example: When shopping, you find exactly what you need, and it's on sale. (I always pray before I go shopping.)

---

31   *The Gift of Miracles*, (Grand Rapids: Inspired, the gift group, Zondervan, 2007), 4.

32   Ibid.

33   Ibid.

We could live our lives unaware and oblivious to the evidences of God's "miracles" all around us. I choose, however, to acknowledge them and to love them, these ordinary, everyday miracles that enrich and bless our lives.

God want us to know that His love itself is the real miracle in our lives. His love is the reason that He meets any needs we bring to Him. He may not always meet them the way we desire, but He will meet them in a way that is best for us. Sometimes He does this though miracles – some big, some small.

Albert Einstein once wrote: "There are only two ways to live your life. One is as though nothing is a miracle, the other is as though everything is a miracle."

My Journal — April 4, 2009

"After James' diagnosis, I prayed every day for miracles: the miracle of healing for James' brain; for health and strength for myself as I cared for him; for protection and wisdom. I know that God's miracles, documented throughout the Bible, occurred to save lives, to demonstrate God's power, to strengthen faith, and to bring healing—physically, emotionally, and spiritually. That is very reassuring to me.

I've never doubted that God is still in the miracle business. That realization was a great comfort in the early days, ten years ago when I desperately needed to know for sure that God was intimately involved in our circumstances. So many times in those days, He lovingly demonstrated His presence in real, practical ways. He still does. Recently, when I was very late for an appointment with our accountant, I could not find an important file that I needed. In desperation, I cried out to God for help, and the missing file fell off a shelf onto my head. You may be laughing. However, I have no doubt that God was visibly affirming His presence with me at that very moment.

James and I have been virtually "homebound" now for over a year. Sometimes I am lonely, and I feel disconnected from life as I once knew and experienced it. Thankfully, at my "lowest point," God will send a "good Samaritan" to our door bearing goodies and so much love. (Lucy)

My Journal — March 27, 2010

"Father, this morning I'm desperate for You. You know that I can't do what You're asking without Your help. It isn't just the thought of giving up what I love so much: This house and much of its contents, our special neighbors, our wonderful church that I can see from where I am sitting, the privilege of being just a few blocks from our middle son, his wife and their boys, the convenience of all my favorite shopping places and doctors. It's also all the unknowns: "Will I have enough physical stamina? Will I have the wisdom this will require?"—and so much more.

Father, I'm asking You for miracles this morning at my Bethel.

> *I'm asking You to reveal the "asking price" for the house. I know You already know it.*

> *I'm asking that the house will sell quickly.*

> *I'm asking that the first people who see it will love it and will buy it for the price I am asking.*

> *I'm asking for supernatural physical and emotional strength and health during the days ahead.*

Father, I'm claiming all of your promises today. In Joshua 1:9, you tell me as You did Joshua, "do not be terrified, do not be discouraged because I will be with you wherever you go" (my paraphrase).

In Haggai 2:5 You made this promise, which I am claiming today: "My Spirit remains among you. Do not fear." Along with David, I will say of You, Lord, "You are my refuge and fortress, my God in whom I trust" (Psalm 91:2). (Lucy)

My Journal — April 3, 2010

"I've been very busy since my last entry that was written in a "valley." While in the valley, I was looking at the impossible task before me and at the pain in my heart. I was doing the "unthinkable": selling my home and moving with James to a Brookdale Senior Living Community, the Hampton at Pearland.

From the valley, I looked at God the Father on the "mountain," and I made a commitment to depend entirely on Him for strength, energy, health, courage and wisdom for this part of our journey. I claimed all of His promises to supply my every need. He already knew what I would need in the next few days. He supplied everything I had asked for—and more—at precisely the right time. That's just like our Father.

On March 28, 2010, I made the final decision to put our house up for sale. I decided to give a friend of our oldest son the opportunity to handle the sale. I knew that he would do an excellent job. I had known and loved him since he and my son were in Kindergarten. Together we decided on the price we should ask. He promised that he would "work harder than anyone else ever would." He began the process by placing a 'For Sale' sign in the yard the morning of March 31.

During the previous three days, I had staged, scrubbed, polished and cleaned every inch of my house. It looked beautiful, making my decision even more difficult. Now, we would wait. We had no idea that the wait would only be fifteen minutes. No, it's not a typographical error. Fifteen minutes after the sign was placed, while my son's friend and I were sitting and talking, a car stopped in front of my house long enough for the woman driver to write down the information on the sign. That afternoon she left a message at his office, requesting to see the house that evening. She said she had been looking for a one-story house in this neighborhood for her parents. Since I had a few last minute things to do and since our yardman was coming the next morning, we decided to have her parents come the next afternoon, April 1. The next morning I dusted, mopped, and cleaned our shower and the oven and microwave.

I got James dressed, and he and I left the house at about five o'clock and went to our son's home nearby for dinner and to wait. Within two hours, our Realtor called with the incredible news that "they loved the house" and wanted it, offering the full price I was asking. It was the amount God had given me.

The most surprising thing about all of this is that I had asked God for miracles: that the first person to see our house would "love it" and would want to buy it for the price I was asking. I had told my Realtor from the beginning that God would sell the house. All we needed to do was trust Him and do our part.

Our faithful Father knew how difficult it would have been to keep the house "perfect" and to be able to leave the house when necessary to show it. All of this would have been so confusing and stressful for James. (And for me.) God is so good. Right now, I'm thanking Him and praising Him with a full heart for His miracles.

During this process another miracle took place in answer to my prayers: I was never tired at the end of those three, long fifteen-hour days. I never had sore muscles, never had trouble getting up at 6:00 each morning after a sleep-deprived night. God truly is Amazing. (Lucy)

∾

A discussion about God's miracles would not be complete without talking about divine healing. I firmly believe that only God performs miracles. I also know that we cannot limit our belief in His miracle of divine healing to our limited, finite understanding.

One of my best friends, Bevo, was a fellow student nurse. After graduation we continued our friendship for years, until her death in 2011, at age seventy-five. While we were still young marrieds, Bevo developed cancer. Even with aggressive treatment, her cancer spread, and she was considered by her doctors at M.D. Anderson Hospital to be incurable. Sitting in church one Sunday, for no reason, she started crying and couldn't stop. She said she wasn't sad. By this point in her illness, her faith had grown tremendously. The next day, Monday, she had an appointment with her oncologist. Standing at her kitchen sink that morning, she surrendered everything to God, her fears, her circumstances, her cancer, her very life. As she prayed, she began to experience a sensation of warmth spreading through her body, from her feet up into her chest and lungs, where the doctors had found a large tumor. She told me that at that moment, she knew that God had healed her. Later that day, when her doctors could find no tumor in her lung, they could only say, "You've had a divine intervention. We have no other explanation."

I'm very sure that this story could be told over and over by many people. I have my story of God's divine intervention in my life. In 2012, I was spending as much time as possible with James who was then living full-time at Clare Bridge. One morning, I discovered a small growth on the right side of my nose near the inner corner of my right eye. I made an appointment with my Ophthalmologist who sent me to the Plastic Surgeon in their office. He diagnosed the growth as a skin cancer that needed to be removed soon because of its proximity to my eye. He scheduled surgery for the next week. On the way home from his office, I prayed and asked God to please heal this small cancer according to His perfect will. James was fragile, and I did not want to be indisposed. Several days went by, and I was very busy with business matters and with my daily visits to James. Two days before the scheduled surgery, I was putting on my makeup when I realized that the growth on my nose was gone. There was no sign on the skin to indicate that anything had ever been there. God performs big and small miracles. Mine could be classed as a small miracle, but it was a miracle, God's answer to a need I had placed at His feet. I had forgotten my prayer, but God had not.

During this same period, my dentist had discovered a tooth that needed a root canal. I prayed about this and asked God for a miracle. When I went in for the procedure, she was shocked that the X-ray showed no indication that this was needed.

Another thing I need to share, before finishing this chapter about God's provision of Miracles, is almost embarrassing to talk about. It's about my miraculous mental and physical health. In spite of the physical, mental, and emotional stress of the past thirteen years, I have "supernatural" health. My doctors are amazed. They tell me that they've never seen anyone my age who has no health problems. My Health Insurance Company loves me. It has been at least four years since I have even had a "cold." I take no medication of any kind. I never have a headache or any other pain, any indigestion or other intestinal problems. I take highly rated vitamins, daily, along with Calcium with D. I eat very wisely and exercise daily as much as I can while sitting and writing, sometimes eight to ten hours a day.

I believe that God has given me this amazing health because He wants me to finish this story, His and mine, the story of His faithfulness during a very long, difficult journey with Alzheimer's disease.

In *My Utmost for His Highest*, Oswald Chambers shares his incredible insights into the issue of health and wellness. I have spent a portion of every day for the past nine years with this book, which has had a profound effect on my life. The wisdom that Oswald Chambers shares through the daily devotionals is incredible and life changing. In the devotional for December 4 he writes: "Health is the balance between the physical parts of my body and all the things and forces surrounding me. To maintain good health, I must have the sufficient internal strength to fight off the things that are external. If I have enough inner strength to fight, I help to produce the balance needed for health. The same is true of the mental life. If I want to maintain a strong and active mental life, I have to fight... Morally it is the same. And spiritually it is also the same. Jesus said, "In this world you will have tribulation, but be of good cheer, I have overcome the world" (John 16:33). I must learn to fight against and overcome the things that come against me, and in that way produce the balance of holiness. Then it becomes a delight to meet opposition. Holiness is the balance between my nature and the law of God as expressed in Jesus Christ."[34]

Several years ago I wrote in my journal a quote by Joni Eareckson Tada: "Faith means believing in realities that go beyond sense and sight. It is the awareness of unseen divine realities all around you."

Will there be miracles as we continue our journey? I don't know, but I will keep praying for these and watching for them. Will God reveal Himself in our circumstances when we seek Him? Yes. Of that, I have no doubt. I will remember that God's love itself is the real miracle in my life. I will gratefully experience miracles in my life, but I will trust the Miracle Maker and worship Him—not the miracle.

~ Never Ending Love ~

A love that never fails. "Hard to imagine, isn't it? Has human love ever failed you? I guess your answer may be, 'Yes it has, more times that I would like to think about.' 1 Corinthians 13:8 promises that 'love never fails.' Not God's kind of love, anyway."[35]

"Love." The very sound of it makes me feel warm and safe. The very thought of it makes me remember cookies and hot chocolate; soft cuddly blankets; my Daddy's lap; family group hugs and sing-alongs; Mother kissing me and tucking me in bed each night; trips to my

---

34 *My Utmost for His Highest*, An Updated Edition in Today's Language, Oswald Chambers, Edited by James Reimann, (Grand Rapids, Discovery House Publisher, 1992), December 4.

35 From *Come Thirsty: No Heart too Dry for His Touch,* by Max Lucado, Publisher Thomas Nelson, October 3, 2006.

Mamaw's for Christmas and the love and wonderful smells that greeted us there.

"Love." Just looking at this four-letter word makes me think of the first time I saw James' reflection in a mirror, a reflection I "fell in love with" before I knew who he was. It was a love that "made my world go round" for fifty-six years and, even now, sustains me.

"Love." This word took on a whole new meaning the first time I held each of my babies and grandbabies. It consumed me; it changed me; it enlarged my world. Even now, those grown-up "boys" hold an enormous part of my heart and add meaning to my life.

"Love." What is its origin? God. God is love. That's it, pure and simple, but yet, profound.

I feel humbled and totally inadequate to write about God's provision of "Love." In the concordance of my Bible, there are four pages of scripture references dealing with God's steadfast, never-ending, unconditional, unfailing love for His people. Because God is love, He brings this provision with Him as he daily walks with us on this difficult journey as caregivers to our loved ones with Alzheimer's.

God's love is beyond human comprehension. The apostle Paul describes for us the "extravagant dimensions of Christ's love." He writes, "Reach out and experience the breadth. Test its length. Plumb the depth. Rise to the heights. Live full lives, full in the fullness of God." (Ephesians 3:18-19, *The Message*). God's love goes on forever. It is never-ending. And, it is immeasurable. As we deal with the burdens and the loneliness of caregiving, nothing is more needed or comforting than knowing that God loves us and walks with us all the time.

Almighty God, the Creator of the universe and everything in it, has written, through His divinely chosen scribes, the most beautiful love story we will ever read. This story about the Lover of our souls is found in the Bible, the greatest book ever written, the world's best-seller every year. Throughout its pages, from *Genesis* through *Revelation,* we see the story of God's love unfolding—God's "Love Letter" to us.

The greatest evidence of God's profound love is found in a baby boy, born in a manger in Bethlehem: God Himself stepping down from His throne in Heaven to take on human form and to live among men on earth. Sin had separated us from God, but through Jesus, He gave us a bridge back to Himself. There are no words to adequately describe the depth of God's love expressed through the birth of His Son. Without Jesus, we would have never known about God's never-ending, eternal love. It is a love so amazing that it prompted Him to allow Jesus to die on a cross as an atonement for our sins. God the Father then raised Him from the dead to save us, to love us, to walk with us, and to be our burden-bearer. Through Jesus, God and 'love' are forever linked.

~ God's Love Is Perfect ~

This unique, one-of-a-kind, perfect love of God does not depend on anything that we do for Him, regardless of what we've been taught or have believed in the past. Jesus has already done it all. We only need to realize and admit that we can do nothing. Our part is to trust and believe what Jesus did on the cross for us and then rest in His perfect love.

I love this statement by Max Lucado, "Does this thought comfort you? It sure comfort's me. God's love does not depend on ours. The abundance of our love does not increase His. The lack of our love does not diminish His. Our goodness does not enhance His love, nor does our weakness dilute it. What Moses said to Israel is what God says to us: "The Lord did not choose you and lavish his love on you because you were larger or greater than other nations, for you were the smallest of all nations. It was simply because the Lord loves you" (Deuteronomy 7: 7-8 NLT).[36]

As I'm writing today on February 8, 2008, I'm thinking about Valentine's Day, which is coming soon. It is a day that brings back memories of Valentine parties at school where we exchanged Valentines with our classmates. Each year, my wonderful artistic mother helped me decorate my "mailbox" to take to the party and she always had extra Valentines for those students who might not receive any.

February 14 is also a day that brings thoughts of love and the anticipation of gifts of love from our "special one." I think I must have every Valentine James ever gave me. Some from the early years of our

36   *Unfailing Love*, Max Lucado, UpWords,—Week of November 20-26, 2002, Copyright (Thomas Nelson).

courtship and marriage are stored in a very large, red, heart-shaped candy box. I'm grateful now that I am, in some ways, a romantic pack rat.

This morning, I've been reading an article by Charles Stanley in the February 2008 *In Touch* magazine. In it, he reminds us that "the greatest gift our heavenly Father has to offer is the one some people have the most difficulty receiving: the gift of His love." He gives two reasons why some struggle with accepting this "excellent blessing." First, something in their past makes them feel undeserving of God's love; they don't feel worthy.

Second, they are disappointed with their circumstances, and they blame God. As a caregiver facing the endless, unthinkable tasks, the sadness and loneliness that make up my days, I can understand that it could be easy for some to believe that God's love is conditional. It would be tempting at times for them to feel that God has turned His back on them and their struggles. The simple truth is that God's love never fails, and it never gives up on us. God's love endures forever; it does not have an expiration date.

Later in the article, Dr. Stanley shares a personal experience. He says there was a time in his life when he was overwhelmed, and he couldn't understand why God had allowed such pain in his life. His "agony was too great" to handle by himself and, in his distress, he cried out to God. Suddenly, he sensed God draw near. (He's telling <u>my</u> story.) It was as if he heard the Lord say, "My love is perfect, and you can trust Me." With that reassurance, he felt his burden lifted and his anxiety fading. He says that at that moment his "understanding of God's love took a huge step forward."

The same God who spoke to Dr. Stanley's heart that day says to our hearts, "No matter what you are going through, I'm going through it with you. I am always with You, and My love for you is "perfect." God's perfect love "drives out fear" (1 John 4:18).

God's love surpasses any other and is so all consuming that it reaches the end of the earth and the depths of our hearts. It has no beginning and no end. It is never-ending. And it is perfect.

~ God's Love Is Unconditional ~

My Journal — April 6, 2008

"Father, this has been a hard day. I was irritable with James, frustrated because he left black newsprint ink all over the kitchen counters and on a new sofa pillow. He loves to read the daily newspaper, over and over and over. He is so precious, and he would never purposely do anything to make my life harder. But You already know that. Please forgive me when my attitude "stinks," and I'm not very lovable. This seems to happen when I'm tired, and I let down my defenses. Even when I'm stumbling, which I do when I take my eyes off You, You still love me unconditionally. Thank You.

Thank You for holding me and for loving me so extravagantly with a love that doesn't depend on my responses to my circumstances. Thank You for never beating me up. When I do give in to grief and "pity parties," I feel You lovingly wiping away my tears, holding my hand, and loving me with a love that never fails, even when I do." (Lucy)

My Journal — September 20, 2009

"I'm learning that nothing is more perfect, more trustworthy, more unconditional than God's unique one-of-a-kind love. I've just read an excellent illustration of God's unconditional love in the "Parade" Section of today's Houston Chronicle. Jeff Foxworthy, TV game show host (Are You Smarter Than a 5th Grader?), and a devout Christian, writes:

"The most important lesson I have learned from my kids is that they have given me a small glimpse of how God must feel about us. Other people may be capable of doing something to destroy your love for them, but your kids can't.

It doesn't mean that you don't get angry or frustrated with them, but you cannot __not__ love them. They're an awesome gift. And I kind of think that's how God looks at us, like, 'Oh, good grief, you're so stupid; you're driving me crazy, but I still love you.'"

Well, Jeff, I'm pretty sure God never calls us 'stupid', and I don't think that we 'drive Him crazy.' But I do know this: God is love, and He is not capable of __not__ loving us. That would not be in His nature. This is such a comforting truth. We have a Father who is 'head-over-heals' in love with each of us, who is passionate about us. His love is 'tailor-made' for each of us.

Probably the most familiar, most quoted verse in the Bible is John 3: 16: "For God so loved the world that He gave His one and only Son, that whoever believes in Him shall not perish but have eternal life."

Max Lucado calls '3:16' the numbers of 'Hope.' I call them the numbers of "Unconditional Love." When we substitute our name for the words 'the world' and 'whoever', this promise becomes a personal love letter to each of us, our guarantee of eternal life with the Father who will never not love us." (Lucy)

God's Love Overcomes:
It Makes the Impossible, Possible

My Journal — Valentine's Day, 2012

"Beloved, love is more than a 'word.' It is more than just a feeling. "True love is neither physical nor romantic. It is an acceptance of all that is, has been, will be and will not

be" (America Online, Tuesday, October 26, 2004). This statement defines the love of an "ideal" caregiver.

We can all acknowledge that there is no emotion greater than the love that comes from God. His love is a part of his very nature. It is sacrificial, completely unselfish love that always thinks of others. It is a love that overcomes all obstacles. When we display this kind of love in our relationships, we are the most like Jesus.

This is the kind of love that my husband demonstrates in his life every day, even in his dementia. After almost thirteen years with Alzheimer's, his love for others has only grown stronger and more evident. I believe that this is because there are no hidden motives or agendas connected with his love. His love for others is entirely unselfish; God's love shines out of him like a beacon of light wherever he is. James' love is a love that has overcome the enemy, Alzheimer's. It overrides and supersedes the dementia that tries, without success, to rob him of his faith, his joy, his gratitude and praise for God's blessings.

It is fascinating to watch James interact with people, whoever they are. I believe that if the President of the United States walked by, James would motion him over, squeeze his hand until it turned "purple", and tell him, "you're too wonderful to be real." Before we sold our home in Pasadena to move to the Hampton at Pearland, I would take James with me to the Walgreens Drug Store near our home. I would park in the "Handicap parking" space in front of the doors, and sometimes I would leave James in the car for a short time. The girls who worked there loved him and they would take turns going out to check on him and to hear him ask them, "Have you always been that pretty?"

One day when I returned to the car, James opened his car door and got out. It was then that I noticed a shabbily dressed, unshaven, elderly man standing, with his head down, on the sidewalk near the entrance. Spellbound, I watched and listened as James walked up to him, stuck out his hand and said, "I'm James Dishongh. What's your name?" Watching *the man's transformation was an unforgettable experience. He lifted his chin, hesitantly stuck out his right hand, looked at James and smiled a toothless smile. They shook hands like old friends, holding one another's hand a little longer than was normal as if not wanting to let go of this "magic" moment. James then reached into his back pocket and pulled out his billfold, as if it were something that he did every day. He took out two one dollar bills, (that's all I kept in there), handed them to the man, patted him on the shoulder, and walked back to the car. The man was still standing there, smiling through his tears, as we drove off. I looked at James and, smiling through my tears, I said, "Honey, what a beautiful thing to do." James said, "God told me to do it because I'm so blessed." (Lucy)*

I'm very aware of the fact that I am incredibly blessed to be married to my sweet James. I know that many of you are caring for loved ones who, because of their dementia, have become angry, mean, unreasonable and often unrecognizable "strangers." James and I have a minister friend whose eighty-five year old mother developed Alzheimer's shortly after James was diagnosed. In her dementia, she cursed, using language that broke his heart. He told me, "I didn't know that my sweet mother even knew those words. I can hardly stand to hear them come out of her precious mouth." Also, his mother often raved and screamed and sometimes threw things at her loved ones when they visited her in the hospital where she was living. Even with medication, she had become a "stranger" to her family, whose hearts were already terribly wounded by her illness. Only occasionally did they get a glimpse of the loving mother and grandmother she had once been. The love and patience required to deal with this kind of "unthinkable" situation can only come from God. In their own strength this dear family could never have endured this tragedy, this loss of their "spiritual Matriarch." How does one deal with someone who has become so "unlovable?" Someone you have always dearly loved and who has loved you?

This friend and I talked about this many times during the last, long, difficult months of his mother's life. Each time we talked, we agreed that God specializes in the "impossible", and that God's grace is the only thing that makes "impossible love", possible. We both acknowledged that the Holy Spirit who lives within us can and will produce the kind of love and patience he and his family needed. We prayed for this each time we talked. When God, in His mercy, took this "saint" home to heaven, I rejoiced with our friend.

Your situation may not be this extreme, but I know from experience, it is never easy. No matter who you are or what turns your life has taken on this strange journey with Alzheimer's, never forget: God is aware of you. In Jeremiah 31: 3, He says, "I have loved you with an everlasting love." As you face each day (and night), if you ask Him, He will draw you close to Himself. His love is already reaching out to you. As I wrote earlier, "This is love, not that we loved God, but that He loved us and sent his Son as an atoning sacrifice for our sins" (1 John 4:10).

Anytime you are feeling alone and overwhelmed, think about the love God has for us—the greatest gift, the greatest provision we will ever receive. It is a gift that will sustain us through our most difficult, loneliest days and nights. It is a gift that keeps on giving. A gift that enables us to overcome all obstacles, even "the impossible." A true test of love is:

✝ To be able to act lovingly even when we don't feel like it;

✝ To be motivated by something deeper and more profound than our feelings;

✝ To act because something deep inside us compels us to reach out with concern, compassion, and love.

Dear God,
Thank You for Your never-ending Love:
A love that is perfect
A love that is unconditional
A love that overcomes
A love that makes "impossible love" possible.

~ Omnipotent Protection ~

Storms are an inevitable part of our lives. Those of us who live near the Gulf Coast are well acquainted with storms that occur in nature. Those of us who care for a loved one with Alzheimer's are well acquainted with a different kind of storm. This storm, like storms in nature, can knock us off our feet, toss us around, and wash us out to sea. It can destroy the things we treasure and disrupt our homes and the normality of our lives. Thankfully, we have a God who rides out our storms with us.

Sometimes, on a clear day, the sun may suddenly disappear behind a black cloud. Then the skies open and the hard rain comes down in a sudden unexpected storm. Our unexpected "storm" was the diagnosis, "Alzheimer's." This "storm" hit hard and left lots of debris and damage. Only our faith in God sustained us for the next thirteen years.

During these years, I've had my share of storms, most of them the result of stress, anxiety and exhaustion. But I've always had an Anchor to hold me and a Safe Harbor to which to run. In God's Word, the prophet Nahum tells us, "The Lord is good, a refuge in time of trouble. He cares for those who trust in him" (Nahum 1:7). Jesus Himself tells us, in John 16:33, "In this world you will have trouble. But take heart. I have overcome the world."

I want to share with you an entry from my journal, written during a time on our journey when I was facing long, dark, lonely nights and raging seas of physical exhaustion. It was the tenth year of our journey with Alzheimer's, the year I discovered that God's omnipotent love was the anchor that held me steadfastly, in spite of the storm that raged around me.

My Journal — March 18, 2009

"I'm at my Bethel on a dark, stormy morning. Thunder and lightning and hard rain woke me very early. James was restless during the night, but he is sleeping soundly for

now. Although the wind is blowing, the rain has slowed to a gentle, intermittent shower. I love storms as long as I'm safely inside. I love to see God's power unleashed in thunder and lightning and wind. His Word tells me that He is in the storm, riding on the clouds. Psalm 104:3 tell us: "He makes the clouds His chariot and rides on the wings of the wind." I love, love, love that mental picture.

Our oldest son loves the ocean. Since his teens, he's always been happier on a surfboard than anywhere else. When the surf's up he wants to be there. He has fearlessly and enthusiastically surfed some of the best surf spots in the world. Oswald Chambers, in My Utmost for His Highest, describes this perfectly: "Huge waves that would frighten an ordinary swimmer produce a tremendous thrill for the surfer who has ridden them."[37]

I have never quite understood how I, the consummate "non-risk-taker," can have such an offspring. The only water in which I feel safe and comfortable is the water in my spa bathtub. I always want to be able to see my feet whenever I'm in water of any kind. I do, however, love to stand on a pier at Galveston and watch and listen as the waves crash over the rocks. There is something powerful and majestic about ocean waves, especially before a storm.

It is rather interesting that I have been reading and studying Psalm 107 this week during my quiet time. The common thread that runs through the Psalm is the feeling of helplessness that the Psalmist is describing. As the Lord's redeemed people encountered trouble of any kind, they eventually "cried out to the Lord in their trouble, and He delivered them from their distress" (Psalm 107: 6).

---

37   *My Utmost for His Highest,* An Updated Edition in Today's language, Oswald Chambers, Edited by James Reimann, (Grand Rapids, Discovery House Publishers, 1992), March 7.

When Alzheimer's disease moved into our lives like a hurricane, it destroyed any control James and I had over our plans and dreams for the future. The destruction left behind was devastating, leaving us feeling entirely helpless. Our first response was to cry out to the Lord and "He saved us from our distress."

One of the troubles that God's people faced in Psalm 107 was the peril of storms. In this Psalm, the psalmist paints a vivid picture of ships being tossed about by storms. The sailors cried out to the Lord, and "He stilled the storm to a whisper; and the waves of the sea were hushed. They were glad when it grew calm, and He guided them to their desired haven" (v. 29-30).

Could it possibly be true that the same God who calms our storms sends storms into our lives for His divine purpose? Everyone will encounter a storm at some time in their life. Storms can be in the form of tragedy, sickness, suffering, losses such as divorce, bankruptcy, death, failures, regrets and disappointments.

Sometimes my storms are brief and do little damage. They are usually caused by the everyday stresses and the unavoidable drudgery of caring for James. Every day is filled with "hundreds" of questions or sometimes, one question asked a "hundred" times. Once, a friend offered to sit with James for a couple of hours. When I returned home, he said, "I didn't know anyone could ask that many questions in two hours."

It is hard to ask anyone to sit with James because he can't always find his way to the bathroom. As a result, he often has "accidents." I've learned to expect and deal with these, but it never gets easier. In caring for all of James' physical and emotional needs, running a household, shopping, managing and keeping various doctor's appointments, I often neglect taking care of my needs. When this happens, my little storms sometimes develop into major "hurricanes."

As much as I love James, the daily stress and strain of being his full-time caregiver often leave me feeling tossed about;

battered and beaten; my sails tattered and torn. These are times I need an anchor, a safe haven, a place of rest and refuge, a shelter in my personal storms. In desperation, I head for my Bethel, and my Father, my Safe-Harbor-God, meets me there. He comforts me, reassures me, and meets all my needs. He says to my storm, "be still." He gently reminds me that there will be other storms in the future, but that He will always be with me. Therefore, I can trust Him and take refuge in that blessed assurance.

"Omnipotent Father, You are my strong tower, my hiding place, my shelter. Thank you for hovering over me no matter how fierce the storm, how loud the thunder, how close the lightning, how strong the wind. With You, Father, I can move through and beyond the storms in my life. Amen."
(Lucy)

~ Plans and Purpose ~

The Scrapbook

Some things in my life were so special
I carefully filed them away
To look at and to remember
On a distant, future day.

I carefully recorded these memories
In the scrapbook of my mind
So that the things I treasured most
I could always easily find.

Whenever I sensed that something
Was unusually special or rare
I took a "mind" picture for my book
And placed it carefully there.

Like the first time I saw James
And the wonder of our first kiss,
All the first things that we shared
I didn't ever want to miss.

Our first home, our first vacation
The birth of our three boys
Things that today are priceless,
Sweet memories of our joys.

Memories of the homes we built
And loved ones who gathered there.
Each home we dedicated to the Lord,
A refuge for us and others to share.

I have special memories of our "dream home,"
The one on Rainbow Bend
That Season of our life, though not perfect,
I never wanted to end.

When one day God said so clearly,
"Lucy, it's time to move away,"
My "blue, white and yellow" memories
Were stored in my book that day.

Although God's words at that moment
I didn't fully understand
I knew that what He had in store
Were changes He had thoughtfully planned.

Some memories of that Season
Are not always comforting or kind,
But I faithfully and carefully stored them
In the corners of my mind.

Like the last time at my "Bethel"
In that house too dear to sell.
Perhaps God knew that I'd begun
to love temporal things too well.

Just as Seasons always change
As God the Creator plans
So also the Seasons of our lives
Are held in His loving hands.

~Lucy

I'm so grateful that God has provided insight into His plans and purpose for this difficult, often confusing season of our lives. I believe that He drew the blueprints for His plans for me with the same hand that created the world.

In the eighth year of our journey with Alzheimer's disease, God gave me a vision for this book, this story of our journey into "alien country," where we often felt like foreigners. We desperately longed to go back to the familiarity of our safe, secure, predictable life. When I realized that there was no going back, I turned to God to guide me and to teach me how to survive in this new world called Dementia.

Although James and I had a strong faith in God our Father, we still experienced the heartache and pain of adjusting to this "New Normal" that was now our life. As we began to walk this unfamiliar path, we turned to God, our "guide," who already had a complete itinerary for our journey. He had planned this season of our life long before we were born. Through His prophet, Jeremiah, He gives us this precious promise: "For I know the plans I have for you, declares the Lord, plans to prosper you and not to harm you, plans to give you hope and a future" (Jeremiah 29:11). Although these words were spoken to the exiled Israelites in Babylon, they spoke directly to my situation and to my heart, and I claimed them.

If I didn't know it before, I soon discovered that we serve a Purpose-Driven God who has a special plan and purpose for each of His children.

James and I made a commitment to God on July 22, 1999, the day his doctor said, "It's Alzheimer's." We promised that no matter how difficult our life might become, we would continue to trust God and look for His blessings. We were committed to focusing on His purpose for us rather than on the problems looming before us.

After the doctor's diagnosis, things began to change rapidly. On his recommendation, we sold our much loved two story house and, in November of 1999, we moved into a new one-story house. It was in a wonderful subdivision behind the church we would join within the next year. Leaving our previous church where we had worshiped, raised our sons, and served for forty years, in many capacities, was not easy, but it was part of God's plans. I came to love our "miracle house" and our new church.

I was learning that when life doesn't go according to our plans, we can either accept God's plans, or we can find a detour. I'm no dummy. So I chose God's plans, even though I didn't always understand. I was learning that true surrender goes far beyond common sense.

In March of 2010, through the concerns of our children and through His Word, God said, "Lucy, it's time for me to reveal the next part of My plans for you and James."

As those plans unfolded, I wanted to cry out, "Please, Father, not that. Are you sure? Isn't there some other way?" But the Holy Spirit reminded me that the Lord's plans are always best, that they would not harm me but would "give me hope and a future."

Therefore, in obedience, I put my "dream home" on the market, (it sold in fifteen minutes), had the "world's largest garage sale," and moved with James to a Brookdale Senior Living Community, the Hampton at Pearland. God the Father already knew that their Memory Care program at Clare Bridge is one of the highest rated programs in the nation.

As part of God's divine plan, the Director of the Hampton graciously accommodated our specific needs by converting two adjoining one-room apartments in Building 2 into one large apartment. It consisted of a king-size bedroom, two bathrooms, two large closets, and a combination Kitchenette, Dining Area, and Sitting Room. The maintenance crew had painted the rooms the colors of my previous "dream house."

They even moved the television cable to the opposite side of our Dining Room-Sitting Room to make room for a large pine hutch that I filled with my blue and white china.

With thoughtful selection of the things I love best, I converted those two rooms into the "model apartment" for the community. Only a heavenly Father, who intimately knew what would esthetically bring me joy, could have lovingly planned such a wonderful substitute for what I had left behind. Even though I was traveling the road of adversity with Alzheimer's, God was blessing me with His best.

Many people would have considered my move and my situation a setback, but I knew it was God's perfect plan and design for us at that point of our journey.

As believers we know that Jesus Christ came into our world to save us and to make a difference in our individual lives, but when He asks us to follow Him into uncharted territory, we are suddenly afraid. We want to trust Him and to follow Him, but we keep encountering "obstacles" and doubts. We often feel like outsiders and strangers in our "new normal." That's when we need to remember to leave room for Jesus, wherever we find ourselves.

God's plan from the beginning of this journey was to give us hearts that would trust Him; hearts in tune with His; hearts that would not lose hope, even in the gathering darkness of Alzheimer's dementia.

Sometimes we no longer can remember what we were like before the stress and busyness of caring for our loved one pushed everything else aside. However, we must never get too busy for quiet times with the Lord through prayer and Bible Study. Now more than ever we need the strength and nourishment we will find there. These times help us to remember that nothing is too hard for the Lord, and that He always holds out the promise of His constant presence with us.

As we spend time with Him, we will discover that He is a "familiar" Friend. As our purpose-driven Lord, He is constantly in the process of working out His purpose in us. He doesn't ever change. Therefore, we can confidently learn to adjust our plans to line up with His, which are much better than ours.

Before Alzheimer's moved into our lives, James and I were content. We had such high hopes, dreams, and plans for our "golden years." Then the reality of what we were facing and of what the future held left us feeling like foreigners transported unexpectedly to an "alien country."

After we moved to Assisted Living at the Hampton, at times my heart desperately yearned for the beauty and the familiarity of our much loved home and life. But as I said before, those doors were closed. That life was gone. There was no turning back. My only choice was to trust God and to learn to love my "new normal" at The Brookdale Community, the Hampton at Pearland. This wasn't always easy because I longed to know the outcome which at times was blurred and hazy. My once predictable life was turned upside down. The future was frightening. I longed for a Burning Bush.

As time passed in this our new "Hampton Season," God began showing up in ways that demonstrated His primary purpose for me, "that you may know that I am God." That verse, Psalm 46:10, "Be still and know that I am God," became the lifeline that He threw out for me anytime I was "lost in my wilderness and storms."

✝ Anytime I felt that I was forgotten, God showed up.

✝ Right in the middle of my hopelessness and loneliness, God showed up.

✝ When my heart grieved over the loss of the person James had been and was no more, God showed up.

Even now, as I face the future without James, learning to live in a world without him, God shows up. He reminds me that He is the One who said in Revelation 21:5, "I am making everything new." Now, when I don't always understand the purpose of His plan, I know that I can trust that His purpose and His plans will "prosper me and not harm me." Because I intimately know the One who made that promise in Jeremiah 29:11, I can confidently step into this new Season, "Life after Alzheimer's."

~ Promises ~

"God's promises stream through the clouds in our soul, bringing strength and the reassurance that this life is but a stepping stone to something far better than we can ever imagine."[38]

I am so thankful that God the Father has packed His promises for our journey. This provision is so important in today's world where there are so few absolutes; so few things we can rely on or trust. It is only in God's Sovereignty and His promises that we find absolute truth, something solid we can stand on as we travel a difficult, sometimes dark path.

There are hundreds of God's precious promises in the Bible. When I pray them back to God, making them the cry of my heart, I find a firm foundation of strength for my role as James' caregiver. I believe that God has a promise for every need and problem in my life, and I believe that He keeps every promise.

The Psalmist wrote these words in Psalm 119:49, "Remember what you said to me your servant – I hang on to these words for dear life. These words held me up in bad times; yes Your promises rejuvenate me" (*The Message*).

Fellow caregiver, looking back over the past eleven years, I realize that my life would have been hopeless without God's promises that are scattered so liberally throughout His Word. Even now, facing what seems to be a never-ending journey, life would be almost unbearable without His promises that daily pour hope into my heart. One example of hundreds is: "Cast your cares on the Lord and he will sustain you; he will never let the righteous fall."

Another one of my favorites is found in Isaiah 41:10: "So do not fear for I am with you; do not be dismayed for I am your God. I will strengthen you and help you; I will uphold you with my righteous right hand." Verse 13 reads: "For I am the Lord, your God who takes hold of your right hand and says to you, do not fear; I will help you."

---

38   (A verse on a Sympathy Card I received after James' death in September 2012 – Author Unknown)

God's promises are precious to me because they remind me that He is present in my world. He is always thinking about me and my needs, my hopes, my dreams. In return for His personal concern for me,

✝ I will place my faith, hope and trust in Him,

✝ I will be obedient to His commands,

✝ I will patiently wait for His perfect plan for me.

When I have done these three things, then I can claim His promises with confidence. I believe that God has brought us to this point in "our story" for such a time as this: To show that He is faithful; that His will to change my world is relentless. This belief gives me the determination to live out "our story" in accordance with His plans and purpose. When I am tempted to take things into my own hands, I will remember Abraham's wife, Sarah. She grew tired of waiting for God's promise to give her a child, and she began to question that promise. When she decided that she knew best, her decision had lasting consequences that have adversely affected many generations to come. Then God, in spite of her lack of faith, fulfilled His promise to her in His perfect timing.

There are some questions we need to ask ourselves to see if a particular promise applies to our situation:

✝ Is this promise limited to a particular person or circumstance, or does it apply to me? An example of this is the story of Sarah in which God's promise to her was specific for her situation.

✝ Am I asking God to meet my need or my desire? An example of my need would be the assurance that God will never forsake me, that when I am exhausted He will hold me with His strong right hand.

✝ Does the fulfillment of this promise require anything on my part? An example would be the promise in James' life verse: Proverbs 3:5-6, "Trust in the Lord with all your heart and lean not on your own understanding; in all your ways acknowledge him, and he will make your paths straight." My part is to trust in the Lord, even when I don't understand.

When we have taken these steps, we can ask confidently for the Lord to fulfill His promises, according to our needs. Hebrews 10:23b reminds us that "he who promised is faithful," referring to the hope we have in our salvation through the shed blood of Jesus Christ. 1 Corinthians 1:20 says, "No matter how many promises God has made, they are "Yes" in Christ."

Before I finish this chapter on "Promises" I want to share some wonderful promises in Proverbs 10. They tell me that, if I am righteous:

✝ I will not die (Proverbs 10:2)

✝ My needs will be met (Proverbs 10:3)

✝ Blessings will fill my life (Proverbs 10:6)

✝ My memory will be a blessing (Proverbs 10:7)

✝ The desires of my heart will be granted (Proverbs 10:24)

✝ I will be planted in the storms of life, and I will still be standing when the storm passes (Proverbs 10: 25, 30)

✝ I will have joy in my life (Proverbs 10:28)

✝ God will protect my life. (Proverbs 10:29)

A great illustration of God's promise of protection in our lives is a story about a young Indian boy who, as part of his Rite of Passage, had to stand in the center of a circle in the woods all night long in the darkness. The possibility of dangerous wild animals filled his mind.

Outwardly he was brave, but inwardly he was terrified. He staunchly made it through the night, exhausted and longing for daylight. When dawn finally came, the boy was surprised to see his father standing just outside the circle with a bow and arrow in his hand. He had been there all through the night, protecting his son.

I love this story, this boy, this father, this truth about my Heavenly Father's love, so beautifully illustrated here. And I love you, dear fellow caregiver. I'm asking God to help us realize that His promises are worth waiting for, that His plans for us are perfect, and that His love for us is inexhaustible and immeasurable.

I want to say, in closing, that I believe James' Alzheimer's has been slowed by the wonderful drug Aricept, but our faith, strength, joy, hope, and courage on this journey have been propelled by God's promises.

> "Affirm your promises to me—promises made
> to all who fear you. Let your love God, shape
> my life with salvation exactly as You promised"
> (Psalm 119:38, 41 *The Message*).

~ Quiet Times ~

I believe that firmly planted in the heart of every believer is a longing for a deeper, more profound, intimate relationship with God. This is because our hearts were designed by our Creator, our Heavenly Father, who wants this relationship with us more than we can imagine. This has been His purpose for us since He created us in His image.

Augustine said it better than I can: "Our hearts are restless until they rest in Thee, 0 Lord."

I don't know about you, but I desperately need to know that God is intimately involved in my life as a caregiver, always working out His purpose through my daily circumstances.

In a journal entry on March 1, 2009, I copied a quote by Joni Eareckson Tada from her book about intimacy with God. "Intimacy with

God involves finding footholds and handholds in His character."[39] That reinforced my belief that real intimacy with God is possible only when we know His character and understand His purposes. Remember, God has an eternal perspective on our situations. He never loses sight of us because we are always on His mind. Because He is our Creator, He is carefully working out His plans for our individual lives.

My Journal — May 5, 2005

"At my Bethel this morning, I'm reading one of my favorite Psalms, Psalm 46. Verse ten is highlighted and underlined in my Bible. "Be still and know that I am God.""

This verse tells me that the only way I can get the message God has for me is to be still in His presence as I come here daily. Then as I shut out every distraction, I will experience His presence as I spend time with Him. As I share my feelings, pray, and read His Word (praying Scriptures back to Him), and then listen, He replaces my anxiety with His peace.

As a result of my "stillness", I can know without any doubt that He is God. Father, thank You for this quiet time with You this morning. These sweet moments I spend with You renew my strength and refresh me for whatever lies ahead for James and me today." (Lucy)

---

39   *31 Days Toward Intimacy With God*, by Joni Eareckson Tada, Multnomah Publishers, 2005.

My Journal — September 3, 2009

Today, at my Bethel, I'm thinking about all the minor things that once stressed me.

The last ten years have taught me some excellent lessons about what's important and what isn't. I'm discovering more each day that the sweetest life is a simple life, filled with quiet times with God, times spent with family and friends, and opportunities for serving others as I am able. I have learned that the greatest peace comes from knowing that God is loving enough, wise enough and strong enough to protect me and to supply my every need. Most important of all, God is revealing to me that the most important ministry I will ever have is caring for my precious, godly James, who can no longer care for himself.

There was a time when I would have "pity parties" where I wondered if anyone missed me at church, in the choir, at Women's Bible Study, at Prayer Retreats, at Something Special for Women, and Missions at Night. Then I would be reminded, by the Lord, that I am very blessed. I have precious sons and daughters-in-law, many wonderful friends who do remember and miss me, a Sunday School Class I am honored and humbled to teach each week, and wonderful intimate worship times with the Lord. Before we became "homebound" we never missed anything—and we loved it all: the great fellowship, worship, music, friends, and great food. But as James became more dependent on me for his care—showering, dressing, shaving, feeding, I realized I was exhausted most of the time. I would often forget to eat, and I lost over twenty pounds in just a few months. Today when I was having a precious quiet time with the Lord, His Spirit said, "Lucy, no more striving. Let me do the striving. You just rest in me." Tears filled my eyes and peace filled my heart, and I made a promise to rest in Him. (Lucy)

My Journal — January 14, 2010

Although it's very early, I'm at my "Bethel." I've thanked God for this new day. I've been awake for a while, listening to the silence, enjoying the solitude, this precious quiet time before the day comes rushing in with its busyness, its responsibilities, and its challenges. I listened gratefully as my precious James breathed peacefully, sleeping soundly after a restless night. Then I slipped quietly out of bed, being careful not to disturb him. I quickly made my way down the hall to the Living room and my "blue-chair-Bethel." Here, I will spend priceless "quality" time with my heavenly Father, as all parents and children should.

As I'm thinking about this special time that I spend here with the Lord each morning, I'm remembering the mornings when I was so troubled and heavy-hearted, I almost ran here to find relief from my stress and fears, comfort for my wounded spirit, and strength for my exhausted body. As I opened my Bible each morning, God faithfully spoke to me through His Word and His Spirit, addressing my needs for that day.

As time passed, I developed an intimacy with God that I had never before experienced but something that I had craved. I found myself spending more time just sitting quietly, letting Him speak hope and comfort to my heart. As He pointed out His messages and promises to me in His Word, I began to grow in my knowledge of His character and attributes. For the first time, I understood what had been missing in my personal relationship with God. It was this intimacy that I had sought.

Why had it taken me so long to experience this great gift, this provision from the Lord? Was it because I was so busy "serving Him that I had neglected spending time with Him, getting to know Him better, receiving His power, His guidance, His wisdom for my many "ministries"?

Did I not realize that I could do nothing without divine power given to me by the Holy Spirit? These provisions were always available to me when I took the time to seek them and to receive them. The problem was I didn't always take the time. No wonder I was often stressed and "burned out."

Did I somehow think that I knew all there was to know about God? That I had all the answers? Don't misunderstand. I loved the Lord with all my heart, and I loved serving Him through my ministry to others. And I prayed. Oh, how I prayed. But my "quiet times" were not exactly "quiet." I did most of the talking—pouring out my heart, laying my request before God, sharing my personal needs.

Each morning I prayed for protection and blessings for James and our children. I prayed for family and friends. I prayed for our church and all the pastors. I prayed for the missionaries and their needs. I prayed for people in the news, for our country. I prayed every time I heard a siren and for whatever need that represented. If you had asked me about my prayer life, I would have told you that it was strong and healthy. But something was missing.

What was that elusive "something"? I had a personal relationship with the Lord, but not the intimacy that my heart craved. I longed to know Him as a "best" Friend, one who would share with me His secrets and beautiful truths I might never know unless I listened to Him speak them to my heart through quiet times spent with Him.

In Deuteronomy 29:29, Moses tells the Israelites in his last message to them before his death and before they crossed over Jordan into the Promised Land: "The secret things belong to the Lord our God, but the things revealed belong to us and our children forever, that we may follow all the words of this law." The same Lord, the God of Moses, will reveal His truths—truths that belong to me—when I take the time to receive them as I go daily into my "prayer closet, my Bethel," and spend time with Him.

In Psalm 25:14, David tells us: "The Lord confides in those who fear him; he makes his covenant known to them." This verse tells me:

God wants to confide in me daily.

God wants to have discussions with me.

God wants to tell me His secrets.

I want to be sensitive at all times to the presence and power of God, to experience His presence in everything that I do. Like Brother Lawrence, I want to intentionally practice staying in constant communion with God.[40] I can do this as I cook, as I vacuum, as I mop and clean the bathroom (sometimes three or four times a day). I can do this as I help James shower, shave, dress, and in all the ordinary, mundane things of life.

Those of us who follow Jesus Christ know and believe the promise that God, through the Holy Spirit, is with us at all times, but we don't always process that truth in our daily lives. At least I didn't until I desperately wanted this meaningful, intimate relationship with God more than I wanted anything else.

It didn't happen overnight; it took time. But it was worth waiting for. I discovered that during those dark, difficult days and nights, as James' needs increased, the greatest comfort and joy I had was this awesome closeness and intimacy with God. James 4:8 promises: "Come near to God and he will come near to you." I began to discover that every promise from God applied to my life in some way, and I began to personalize them. As God spoke fresh truths into my heart, I realized that He is worthy of my undivided attention at all times. As I began practicing and nurturing this fresh, new relationship with the Lord, I no longer felt the need to be constantly striving. I had found what I had been seeking. Thank You, Father, for this relationship with You, this intimacy." (Lucy)

---

40   Brother Lawrence, *The Practice of the Presence of God*, copyright 1958, 1967 by Fleming H. Revell, (Spire Books, P.O. Box 6287, Grand Rapids, MI.)

❧

Have you ever thought about the fact that God hears our prayers even when we don't verbalize them? That He answers prayers we don't know we've prayed? That every sigh, every heartache is a plea that reaches God's ears?

During this past decade of life with Alzheimer's, I've spent so many hours praying and listening to God speak through His Word, I've learned to recognize His voice. It was when I became a "homebound" caregiver and my problems became God-sized that I learned how to pray. I've learned that after I lay my request before Him, I must be still and listen and wait for His answer. As a "homebound" caregiver, He has my undivided attention.

I had never thought about the fact that Jesus never talked about unanswered prayers. That's because God always answers our prayers. When we get ourselves, our doubts, our skepticism out of the way, we will see God at work. It is only when we fail to take time to listen that we make foolish and sometimes costly mistakes. Wow. That should be a wake-up call to each of us.

So much has been written about prayer, it seems there would be nothing more to say, no new thoughts or insights. God Himself, however, is showing me something new and fresh every day. He is always reminding me that listening to Him is not some casual activity. It is the most important thing I can do for myself, for James, and for others. For example, when I awake suddenly during the night, and a particular person comes to mind, I know that at that moment, I need to pray for that person. This is a wonderful gift that God has entrusted me with, the gift of intercession.

Intercessory Prayer is a ministry I can do at any time, even during these "homebound" years as James' Alzheimer's advances. If I honestly believe that the greatest gift I can give my children and my friends is intentional time devoted to prayer on their behalf, that should take precedence over a multitude of other things that don't matter, but which fill my day.

My Journal — January 25, 2011

"In the middle of all the unsettling changes in my life the past ten months, in my "New Normal," my "Hampton Season," I'm finding simple yet profound truths about myself:

I no longer sweat the small "stuff."

I'm more likely to listen to God, waiting for His instructions.

I no longer need to understand everything that has happened and is happening in my life.

I'm developing a deeper trust and confidence in God, believing that He is still in absolute control, even in this strange season.

I know that no matter how brutally frank my prayers, God will listen and not judge me.

I have come to believe that God accepts my anguished pleas and questions as I verbalize my heartache and loss. I once believed that I had to be careful not to offend God, not to lose my "cool", not to allow my frustrations to surface. Here, in this season, I am learning that when my "venting" is over God is still here, still listening, still loving me.

My first real breakthrough to intimacy with God occurred while I was flat on my face in my closet, begging God for strength to endure the reality of James' Alzheimer's. That was almost twelve years ago, and I'm still asking God for strength to face each long, restless night.

The difference between those days and today is that when I come to God in prayer, I always find a safe, quiet place in His loving presence. Now I realize that God has never left me even for a second in all those years. Because I have come to know Him so well, I know that He will continue to walk with me until this journey with Alzheimer's is over and beyond.

Another difference is that I have become a stronger, more resilient, more trusting, woman of faith. I've reached this point in my journey, not in spite of, but because of the tragedy of Alzheimer's.

I'm writing today from the upstairs balcony across the hall from our apartment at the Hampton. Although the air is cold, the welcome sunshine is warming my spirit. I come here after James is safely next door at Clare Bridge. When the four walls of our two-room apartment begin to close in and my soul yearns for communication with God, I come here to worship Him as He reveals Himself to me through nature. Although this is not where I would have chosen to be, I know that God has chosen this beautiful place for us— this "safe" place. The flowers, the trees, the beautiful grounds of this "new" home nourish my soul and my need for this beauty provided by God. Thank You, Father." (Lucy)

My Journal — April 3, 2012

"I'm sitting in my familiar blue chair, my Bethel, in my "New Normal," the house I had built less than a minute away from Clare Bridge at the Hampton where James now lives full time.

A spiritual reality that continues to thrill me and strengthen me more than any other thing in my life is God's desire to speak to me, just an ordinary woman. This is reality: that Yahweh, The Most High God, wants to meet with me in His "secret place"; He wishes to spend precious time with me, to reveal His secrets to me at my Bethel. In the quietness of this place, in the stillness of each morning, He meets me where He has already prepared a table for me, a "table of inwardness." Here He speaks to my heart and listens to my deepest thoughts and needs and my cup runs over. This God, who has been my Shepherd all of my life, already knows my thought and needs, but He wants to hear them expressed from my heart to His.

On this thirteen-year journey with Alzheimer's disease, God has become my Rock, my Anchor, my Shelter, my Comforter, my Father, my Abba. I talk to Him day and night, thanking Him, praising Him, whispering my needs, fears and anxieties to Him. The most recent, most tangible confirmation that God, who never sleeps, is always listening, even during my long sleepless nights, occurred early one morning several weeks ago. I woke up at 4:55 in a cold sweat and a "deep, black hole." I cried out, "Father, I need You." Suddenly a familiar, much-loved scripture came to mind, "Be still and know that I am God." I could picture the words in my Bible: Psalm 46:10, underlined and highlighted and dated 5/5/05. I began saying the verse over and over, first in my mind, then aloud. At 5:00 I got up and made my way to my "blue chair Bethel," turned on the lamp and randomly opened a small devotional book I keep by the chair with my Bible. There before me were the words God and I had been saying: "Be still, and know that I am God." It was not the scripture for the day, but one God apparently wanted me to see.

I knew, more precisely than I've ever known anything, that God was beside me; had been beside me since I awoke; was speaking those very words to me. I was so moved, so filled with His love and His presence, all I could do was sit quietly in this suddenly Holy place, this hallowed ground. With tears streaming down my face, my heart completely at peace, I began to thank and praise my forever-faithful God, my Father. My heart sang all that day and even now, every time I relive this experience in my mind, I am again thrilled and amazed by such extraordinary, boundless love.

As I'm here at my Bethel, writing these thoughts, I'm asking the Lord for insight to share what I'm learning with you. He wants me to tell you that one of the things He loves most about being our Father is the time we spend with Him, talking and listening to one another.

On a personal note, He wants me to tell you that "all things really do work together for good to those who love the Lord and are called according to His purpose" (Romans 8:28). He wants me to tell you that out of the tragedy and heartbreak of Alzheimer's has come this gift of intimacy with my Heavenly Father that I might have otherwise missed. I can honestly say, "Thank You, Father, for this journey with Alzheimer's." (Lucy)

~ Rest and Relief From Stress ~

Several years ago at a Women's Conference, I bought a shirt printed with the words "Too Blessed to be Stressed." Somehow, I felt empowered when I wore that shirt. Also, I enjoyed watching people's reaction to it. The words on the shirt became a slogan by which I tried to live each day. Anytime I began to feel stressed, I reminded myself that no matter what was happening, God was with me and was blessing me; that I was too blessed to be stressed.

Now, more than ever, I need the message of that shirt as I care for James in what is probably the most stressful period in my life. Thankfully, God has promised rest and relief to those of us who are weary and "heavy laden" with the burdens of caregiving.

We can all agree that stress is a natural part of life in an imperfect world. Even devout Christ followers are not immune. No wonder we're stressed. We live in the world that increasingly offers us less and less to hold on to, little hope for mankind's problems and stress, and no promise of spiritual or emotional rest.

At times, on this journey with Alzheimer's, I feel that things in the world and in my life are spinning out of control. Then God shows up and offers me a place to stand, to rest, to hope. He reminds me that He is the Most High God who is still in complete control of the world, at all times. In His Word, He tells us that He has designed us with the capacity to deal with and even grow because of the stress that plagues our lives.

His timeless Words in Psalm 46:10, "Be still, and know that I am God," were spoken to give us the confidence we need to deal with whatever stress we are experiencing. He knew that actually knowing Him would help us to surrender our stress to Him.

My Journal — November 1, 2007

"I noticed recently, as James and I were walking the short distance down the block to our mailbox, that large cracks were beginning to develop in parts of the sidewalk. I held James' arm, taking extra care that he did not trip or stumble on one of the cracks. Our son explained that these were probably caused by stress due to the shifting of the soil beneath the sidewalk.

As I thought about this, I recalled reading somewhere recently that almost seventy years ago, the Tacoma Narrows Bridge, "Gallopin' Gertie", collapsed into Puget Sound. Open to traffic for only four months, this magnificent structure collapsed due to a design flaw combined with gale force winds. This could have been a deadly mistake, but thankfully it wasn't. It was, however, very costly, and it led to engineers redesigning structures to better withstand high levels of stress.

This story made me aware of the destructive properties of stress in my life. Today, I'm asking the Lord, the Master Designer, to give me extra strength to withstand the devastating effects of caregiving stress and the high winds of change that are blowing into my world." (Lucy)

Even before we learned that James had Alzheimer's disease, we had the normal stress common to all adults. We never had to look for it—it found us. We experienced stress related to health issues. For example, James had a quadruple coronary artery bypass in 1994. We had aging parents, adult children and their problems, decisions about retirement, financial and investment concerns.

With the dreaded diagnosis, "Alzheimer's," affecting everything in our lives, our level of stress increased dramatically. Even though I am a Registered Nurse, I often found myself overwhelmed by the physical and emotional needs of my husband. Because James had always brilliantly taken care of our financial affairs, my knowledge concerning these things was very limited. Just maintaining our car was a stress producer I never expected to face—and the list goes on and on.

In desperation, while floundering in the growing reality of my limitations, I turned to the Lord, who was always "waiting in the wings," ready to step in when I acknowledged my need for His intervention.

In answer to the financial "puzzles", the Lord gave me a "crash course" in money management. He also sent to us an excellent financial advisor.

In answer to my helplessness concerning everything related to our car, the Lord sent to us an "automobile angel." He lovingly and expertly took care of all our "car needs" for the next ten years.

In answer to my physical exhaustion and my need for "perfection," the Lord sent to me a precious friend, who lovingly and efficiently kept my "miracle house" looking perfect.

Of course, the greatest answer to my stress was the Lord Himself who stood by my side, day and night. He already knew the "Ten Warning Signs of Caregiving Stress:"

1. Denial about the disease and its effect on the person who's been diagnosed. I know _____ is going to get better.

2. Anger at the person with Alzheimer's or others: that no effective treatments or cures currently exist, and that people don't understand what's going on. If he asks me that question one more time, I'll scream.

3. Social withdrawal from friends and activities that once brought pleasure. I don't care about getting together with the neighbors anymore.

4. Anxiety about facing another day and what the future holds. What happens when he needs more care than I can provide?

5. Depression begins to break your spirit and affects your ability to cope. I don't care anymore.

6. Exhaustion makes it nearly impossible to complete necessary daily tasks. I'm too tired for this.

7. Sleeplessness caused by a never-ending list of concerns. What if he or she wanders out of the house or falls and hurts himself or herself?

8. Irritability leads to moodiness and triggers negative responses and reactions. Leave me alone.

9. Lack of concentration makes it difficult to perform familiar tasks. I was so busy, I forgot we had an appointment.

10. Health problems begin to take their toll, both mentally and physically. I can't remember the last time I felt good.

Every day, as I faced the reality of my stressful situation, the Lord gave me promise after promise in His Word and so many truths to live by. He reminded me, "Rather than depending on your strength and wisdom, immerse yourself in My promises to you. Until you learn to do this, you will break under the inevitable stress and strain of caring for James."

These are some of my favorite promises from the Lord:

"God is our refuge and strength, an ever-present
help in trouble" (Psalm 46:1).

"My God will meet all your needs according to his
glorious riches in Christ Jesus" (Philippians 4:19).

Of course, the greatest promise and invitation we could ever receive in the midst of our stress is one from Jesus Himself: "Come to Me, all you who labor and are heavy-laden and overburdened, and I will cause you to rest; I will ease and relieve and refresh your souls" (Matthew 11:28 AMP).

The Lord knew that we would need this reminder. He knows that much of my stress in the past came from too much activity and too little quiet time spent with Him. My "servant" heart was eager to serve Him in any and every capacity, but in my busyness, I was neglecting to stay plugged into my power source, God the Holy Spirit.

Now, I needed that power more than ever. I began spending time every morning with the "source", my Heavenly Father. I love the *Psalms*, the Bible's praise book, and I read several of them every morning. The morning after I had noticed the cracks in our sidewalk, I read these very words from one of my favorite Psalms: "The Lord makes firm the steps of the one who delights in him; though he may stumble, he will not fall, for the Lord upholds him with his hand" (Psalm 37:23).

I smiled through my tears as I read these timely, personal words of assurance from my hands-on Father.

I believe that God is always with us and is providing the rest and relief we need in the middle of the stress and strain of caregiving. I believe that He will hold us with His strong right hand and will turn our stress and exhaustion into stepping-stones back to a place of quiet rest with Him. He will be our lifeline when we are emotionally exhausted and overwhelmed by caregiving.

There are also good support services available to us as caregivers. It is important to have a safe forum of understanding people where we can honestly express our frustrations and fears. Caregiver burden, a term often used to describe the stress of caregiving, can be alleviated with the help of a good support group.

Interfaith CarePartners, in Houston, Texas is an educational, non-profit organization that provides wonderful Care Teams and Caregiver Conferences. Also, it places Caregiver Support Groups in many local churches. These groups help those who feel weak and vulnerable from the burden of caregiving and those who feel isolated and alone. I believe these programs are God -inspired. James and I were the grateful recipients of just such a program in our church before we moved to the Brookdale Assisted Living Community in Pearland.

As I've been praying about what else I should share with you, God revealed this to me: "Reasons for Caregiver Weariness:"

1. The length of the journey: It's natural to want to know the outcome, but God doesn't work on our clock or our calendar. Had I known our journey would last for thirteen years, could I have endured? God always knows what's best. Rest in Him.

2. Disappointments: Unmet and unrealistic expectations; broken or unfulfilled dreams. God has a plan. Trust Him.

3. Day to day challenges: Problems and worries can pile up, blocking our view of God. Don't lose sight of God. When He says, "I'll never leave you or forsake you," believe Him.

4. People: Some people have a way of "knocking the wind out of our sails" with their platitudes. They say things like, "If your faith were stronger, you wouldn't be going through this." Et cetera, to ad nauseam. Don't listen to them.

5. Comparison with others: No one's life is perfect, even if it appears to be. It is especially difficult for me to see other

couples, apparently well and happy, traveling and doing things together, living out their dreams. Don't envy others. Be glad for them.

We could all put our own "spin" on these reasons. For example, one of my greatest disappointments has been not having my strong, handsome husband, the love of my life, beside me as I grow old. One of our favorite sayings was: "Grow old along with me; the best is yet to be." I still miss our annual Fall trip to Colorado to see the mountains and the golden Aspens. I regret the trips we planned but never got to take together: An Alaskan Cruise, a trip to the Holy Land, a mission trip to Africa.

I could write another "War and Peace" about the challenges I faced as James' caregiver (but I won't). I will mention a couple: (1) Finding a yardman to handle the mowing, fertilizing, mulching of our lawn while James, the world's most meticulous landscaper and recipient of the Most Beautiful Lawn in the Neighborhood Award, sat at the window, watching him work. (2) Keeping up with all of James' doctor's appointments; picking up and administering medications, keeping them refilled; driving James to the VA Hospital for checkups and lab work.

So far in this chapter, I've discussed the Warning Signs of Caregiver Stress and the Reasons for Caregiver Weariness and Stress. I'd like to close with some practical tips for reducing stress, which I've learned from personal experience.

1. Simplify your life. It took me a long time to do this. I didn't want to give up the things I had always done and which gave me so much joy and satisfaction. For the first seven years of James' illness, I continued to host our large family get-togethers on almost every holiday. I continued to teach a large Single Adult Sunday Bible Study. I continued to be an advisor to the Women's Mission Organization. I sang in the church choirs and a Women's Ensemble. I participated in all the Women's Ministry events, decorating tables for Something Special for Women and Prayer Retreats. I prepared materials for and taught Mentoring Classes for Women at our church. I helped serve lunch to the BSM at the local colleges.

I prepared the Prayer Emphases for Missions at Night, which met once a month. I taught in Vacation Bible School every summer at my church (also, in the early years, at our previous, small church). I did much of this with only four or five hours of sleep. No wonder I was exhausted and stressed.

2. Recognize and accept limits. (Need I say more?) As you can see, I had set unreasonable goals for myself. My striving and perfectionism almost "did me in." The hardest thing for me was "letting go" and learning to say "No." Just do it.

3. Learn to reach out to others for support and to accept their help. The loneliness and isolation that is the result of this "new normal," caregiving, can cause us to become disconnected from the very thing we need most, which is the support of our friends. As we are gradually forced to give up many of our social connections, we begin to feel like an "island." We feel separated from the familiarity of routines of the past group activities, ministries, and friendships. We begin to feel abandoned and we often wonder if anyone misses us or remembers where we are and worse, "if they even care." This experience of "isolation" is real and can be very damaging. However, try to remember that others may not know our needs unless we share them. They have busy lifestyles and responsibilities and stressors of their own. Many of my friends have expressed regrets that they did not realize how much I needed them. So, swallow your pride and ask for help.

4. Get regular exercise. I know, you're probably thinking, "Are you serious? I'm already exhausted." I am serious. The right kind of exercise is relaxing, emotionally and physically. For example, I turned on lively music and danced—sometimes with James—but usually by myself. I learned to "Dance like no one is watching." After my

quiet time with the Lord each morning, I sat on the floor and did Yoga to soothing music. Deep breathing is very relaxing. As I watched a favorite TV show, I often did jumping jacks, walked or jogged in place, or lay on the floor and did leg lifts.

5. Find ways and reasons to relax and have fun. Call a friend to come for coffee or tea. I even called one friend occasionally to pick up lunch and come over so we could spend time together. When I did have an opportunity to spend time with friends, I tended to "talk their arm off." As James became more childlike, I felt like I did as a mother of toddlers—"desperate" for adult conversation. I found it to be extremely helpful to express my "bottled up" stress to caring friends, knowing that they would not judge me for "venting." That's why I've tried to honestly and transparently share with you my frustrations and the ways I discovered to cope with them to reduce my stress.

6. Focus on the blessings, the positives, the joy-bringers. Learn to find satisfaction in simple pleasures: the beauty around you, the love of friends and family, the privilege of caring for your loved one. My love for James and my commitment to caring for him was what gave purpose and meaning to that season of my life. My faith in God gave me the courage and strength that I needed to deal with the inevitable stresses of caregiving. When I focused on God's faithfulness in meeting my needs, my anxiety was eased, and the daily activities of caring for James were often transformed into special moments that gave meaning then and sweet memories for me now.

~ Strength ~

"My grace is sufficient for you, for my strength
is made perfect in weakness"
(2 Corinthians 12:9).

If there is one thing I've discovered on our journey with Alzheimer's, it's this: "Caregiving is not for sissies." That's why our Gracious God has given us the much-needed provision of strength and energy.

The Apostle Paul, while in chains, prayed this prayer for the faithful Christians in Ephesus: "I ask the God of our Master, Jesus Christ, the God of glory to make you intelligent and discerning in knowing him personally, your eyes focused and clear, so that you can see exactly what he has called you to do, grasp the immensity of this glorious way of life he has for Christians, Oh, the utter extravagance of his work in us who trust him —endless energy, boundless strength" (Ephesians 1:18-19, *The Message).*

I love God's Word. I love this prayer from the heart of a man who was in prison when he wrote this letter. He was imprisoned because he was relentlessly faithful to God's calling in his life. His life demonstrates for me that no matter where I am or what I am facing, I, too, can be faithful to God's calling to care for James.

Like Paul, I want to view my circumstances as God's "extravagant work" in me when I place my trust in Him. That "work" includes "endless energy and boundless strength." The words "endless" and "boundless" mean that they can never be used up or depleted.

My Journal — May 24, 2009, 6:00 A.M.

"Father, this morning I'm praying for strength for today. James has a doctor's appointment, and neither of us slept much last night. In Your Word, You have pointed out the truth that my strength is a gift only You can give. It is a gift

for which I am the guardian. You opened my eyes and heart to the fact that you have entrusted me with supernatural strength and energy to take the best possible care of James. Thank You, Father, for this wonderful gift. I will guard it well." (Lucy)

The morning I wrote this journal entry, I was exhausted. James had tossed and turned most of the night, frequently patting or stroking my arm to be sure I was there. Because of Sundown Syndrome, he never feels safe after dark. I often think about how frightening it would be to awaken in the dark and not know who or where you are.

I am so grateful that God is providing the strength that I need to care for James. I feel privileged to have been called by God to serve him and to minister to his needs. James is the love of my life and the most remarkable man I've ever known. It is an honor to be his wife and now his caregiver.

It is amazing that with so little sleep and rest at night, I am infused with strength and energy during the day. During this "Homebound Season" I'm learning to accept eagerly God's daily supply of everything that I need. It reminds me somewhat of the manna God provided for the children of Israel on their journey to the Promised Land. He gave them just exactly enough for each day. They couldn't hoard it, saving it for the future. They didn't need to. As I'm learning more about God's consistent faithfulness, I can trust that He will take care of my needs for today, and then for tomorrow, and for all the days ahead.

To access God's incredible power, we must first recognize and acknowledge our frailty. This reminds me that recently when I was vacuuming the den, I reached down to pick up my grandson's twenty-pound barbells. I discovered to my surprise, that I could not pick them up, no matter how much I tried. This incident revealed to me the truth that I always need my Father's help no matter how strong I feel.

One of the things we will never understand in this life is the divine omnipotence of God and the nature of His power. In simple faith, we can trust God's promise that He will strengthen those who wait for Him. When we do, we will discover that He was here all the time just waiting for us to ask for His help. That is why Jesus said in *Matthew*

11:28, "Come to me, all you who are weary and burdened, and I will give you rest."

Think about it. We can borrow strength from the Lord when our supply runs low. Paul reminds us in Ephesians 3:20, that God "can do immeasurably more than all we ask or imagine, according to his power that is at work within us." This inner strength which God gives us by His power enables us to endure whatever we face as caregiver to our loved one.

When we are exhausted, it would be so easy to give in to despair and discouragement. I'm often tempted to ask, "Does anyone understand or even care about what I deal with twenty-four hours each day? Does anyone understand the pressure and stress of my situation?" When I start to feel this way, I find my Bible and turn to *Psalm 139*.

This psalm tells me that God has a personal, intimate knowledge of every second of my everyday life. His knowledge of me goes far beyond the difficulties I'm facing at any time, day or night. Because of His great love, I am never out of His sight or out of His mind.

Each morning I make this commitment: "I will not be distracted by my physical and emotional exhaustion. I will view this from my Father's perspective:"

✝ He knows that the greatest faith-builder is my awareness of His presence and power in the midst of my exhaustion and despair.

✝ He knows that the best answer to my desperate prayers for help is the realization that He has given to me an inner strength that nothing can steal, not even the endless, exhausting days as James' full-time caregiver.

In her powerful book, *Lioness Arising*, Lisa Bevere, writes: "Allow the Holy Spirit to assess your strength in the light of God's Word, and allow hardship to become a training session, knowing that you will rise from it invincible. Allow the weight of God's Word and the tempering and training of the Holy Spirit to quicken and develop the weak and injured areas of your life. Focus on who you are in your spirit. Don't fear the strength you discover within you. Instead, glorify God with it.[41]

Oswald Chambers, in *My Utmost for His Highest* says essentially the same thing. To quote him: "God does not give us overcoming life. He gives us life as we overcome. The strain of life is what builds our strength. If there is no strain, there will be no strength. If you completely give of yourself physically, you become exhausted. But when you give of yourself spiritually, you get more strength. God never gives us strength for tomorrow, or for the next hour, but only for the strain of the moment."[42]

Jesus Christ tells us in John 16:33, "In this world you will have trouble, but take heart. I have overcome the world."

I believe that God is telling us through all of this that He delivers us "in" our adversity, rather than "from" it. I love that, and I will remember it during the hard times.

❦

All these beautiful truths from God's Word and from gifted, inspired writers, are great and encouraging. But when life gets "real" and we are faced with the "nitty-gritty", (yes, it is a real word, found in *Webster's New Twentieth Century Dictionary)*—the actual, basic facts, elements, and issues of our lives, we need hands-on help; practical answers and solutions.

I am so independent. Also, I am somewhat of a "control freak" at times, something I'm ashamed to admit. I didn't ask for help; I wanted to be the one to take care of James. If I could live the last five years again, I would do things differently. I don't mean that I would not

---

41   *Lioness Arising*, Lisa Bevere, WaterBrook Press, Colorado Springs, Colorado 80921, 2010, p. 76.

42   *My Utmost for His Highest*, An Updated Edition in today's Language, Oswald Chambers, Edited by James Reimann, (Grand Rapids, Discovery House Publishers, 1992), August 2.

still trust God with all my heart and depend on His grace every day. What I mean is I would have had someone come in regularly to sit with James so that I could take a worry-free bubble bath; take a nap; have lunch with a friend; see a movie; go shopping; go walking or jogging.

I'm saying this for those of you who are just beginning your journey with your loved one. I don't ever plan to view my life through a rear view mirror. That would be foolish and a waste of time. However, I always want to share the wisdom God has given me these past few years. That's what we all should do with lessons we've learned from the past.

In Romans 15:1-2 (*The Message*), Paul tells us that "those of us who are strong and able in the faith need to step in and lend a hand to those who falter, and not just do what is most convenient for us. Strength is for service, not status. Each of us needs to look after the good of the people around us, asking ourselves, 'How can I help?'"

The best way to find fulfillment and purpose in our role as caregivers is to realize that it is an honor and a privilege to lend strength to our loved one with dementia and to other caregivers. That's why I call caregiving a "high calling."

When I finish this book—my "War and Peace," as my sons refer to it—I plan to reach out to those who are struggling with the "nitty gritty" of their lives as caregiver to their loved one with this terrible disease. I want them to know that I really do understand how they're feeling and what they're dealing with daily. I want them to know that I have come out on the other side of my journey stronger, more resilient, wiser and victorious.

As I've said before somewhere in this book, "Feel free to borrow some strength from me." I want to be accessible to those who need a "strong friend who's been where they are" for thirteen years. There are probably those who felt sorry for me, "imprisoned" by James' Alzheimer's all those years. But I saw those years as a ministry to James, a testimony of God's wondrous love demonstrated so beautifully in the "utter extravagance of His work in me." It is a perfect picture of God's faithfulness to those who love and trust Him.

Paul said it beautifully: "I'm not saying that I have this all together, that I have it made. But I am well on my way, reaching out for Christ, who has so wondrously reached out for me. Friends, don't get me wrong: By no means do I count myself an expert in all of this, but I've got my eye on the goal, where God is beckoning us onward to Jesus. I'm off and running, and I'm not turning back" (Philippians 3:12-13, *The Message*).

In closing, I want to share this with you: "My gracious Father has for the past thirteen years given me supernatural physical and mental health and wellness. He has also given me endless energy and boundless strength. I'm still experiencing all these blessings every day, even though I'm on the "short side" of eighty years of age. I will always be in awe of such grace."

There were times on my journey that the path was so steep I wanted to give up, but I knew that the "view from the top" would be worth the climb. Therefore, with God's help, I kept climbing. When I was tired or weak because of an unusually steep incline, I would ask Jesus for help, and He would "carry" me. He would tell me, "You can always borrow some strength from Me."

I was right. The view from the top is worth it. However, I know that there is so much more ahead as I continue my "new journey," still keeping the final destination in sight—my "Real Home."

~ Transformation ~

The potential for divine transformation is a provision that God has made available to each person on his or her life journey. Transformation is the goal of God the Creator. It is a process that requires complete submission to the Lordship of Jesus Christ.

Romans 12:2 tells us: "Do not conform any longer to the pattern of this world, but be transformed by the renewing of your mind. Then you will be able to test and approve what God's will is, his good, pleasing and perfect will."

This process of being transformed begins when we ask for it in faith, believing the promises of God in His Word. We are told in 2 Corinthians 3:18: "We, who with unveiled faces all reflect the Lord's glory, are being transformed into His likeness with ever-increasing glory, which comes from the Lord, who is the Spirit."

God the Father wants to become the master potter for every piece of clay He has created. My paraphrase of Romans 12:2 is: "When we are transformed by the renewing of our minds, we will then be able to discover and experience God's perfect will for us."

God's divine transformation takes us from death into life, a new life in Jesus which we enter as newborns—newborns with all the possibilities and potential available to us through our Father God. God's Word tells us in Ephesians 2:10 that, as products of God's workmanship, created in Christ Jesus, we are equipped with special abilities to serve Him. For this reason, the Potter selects not just any clay for each newborn vessel, but the perfect clay for the vessel He wants us to become.

I believe that God knew before we were born that we would be caring for a loved one with Alzheimer's. I also believe that He will mold us into the perfect vessel to serve Him as we serve them. In the process of our transformation, our Father, just as any Potter must do, will knead us, pound us, bend us, shape us, and reshape us until we are "just right." Even though this may be painful and stressful, the end product will be worth it all. Only the Master Potter knows when we are complete.

Because God's purpose is to transform us into the likeness of His Son, Jesus, one of our outstanding characteristics should be the revelation of Jesus' character lived out in us. Like a mirror, we should be reflecting the very nature of God so that others will see Jesus revealed in us. Every day, look in the mirror and say, "I am awesome in Jesus." The role of caregiving gives us the perfect platform to demonstrate God's nature.

Keep in mind that the message of salvation is the most powerful transformation agent in the world. With this knowledge, our desire should be that the glorious message carried around in us—simple vessels of clay—will be spilled out on everyone we meet. My goal is that, as I lovingly and faithfully care for James, I will be making an impact in my world. Also, wherever I go, I want to demonstrate my sincere concern for others by my compassion, my friendless, my smile, my joy. This is a ministry I can do, even as a full-time caregiver.

Sometimes on this journey we feel so battered and worn, it's hard to see the vision that God has for us. Thirteen years ago, before I started my journey with Alzheimer's, a strange, unfamiliar companion, I considered myself a strong, mature Christian. It didn't take me long, however, to realize that I was unfinished, a cocoon—safe, satisfied, protected, and content with my life. At that time, I hadn't been planning or anticipating any significant changes. God, on the other hand, saw my undeveloped potential to become something better, stronger, wiser, more inspiring, and more effective.

He saw inside my safe, complacent cocoon a "butterfly" who could be:

a contagious, effective witness,
a beautiful example of His grace,
a testimony to His greatness,
a perfect portrait of His love.

You see, Psalm 139 tells me that He knew me long before I began this new journey. He knew that, if I would let Him, He would lead me, process by process, to accomplish His purpose for this trial, this "disruptive moment" in my safe, secure life. When I am tempted to look around and compare my life with others, I realize that they, too, have struggles and trials, no matter how perfect their lives appear to be.

God, the Creator, the Master Potter, the Top Chef, doesn't cut corners, doesn't skip steps, doesn't leave out ingredients.

God is very loving, thoughtful, careful and skillful as He works in our lives. He knows that parts of the process of our transformation into loving caregivers are often uncomfortable, even painful and heartbreaking. But He sees the finished product:

the beautiful teapot,
the delicious cake,
the awesome butterfly,
the patient, loving, faithful caregiver.

He sees us as someone who, with His help, will come out on the other side of the process stronger and braver. Our Father knows that for many of us, there will be life after caregiving.

On this journey there will be sweet seasons of life intermingled with bitter, difficult seasons. There will be dry, desert seasons when we will feel temporarily lost in our wilderness of exhaustion and despair. There will be valleys of heartache and grief. It is in the valley that many of us will want to give up instead of waiting patiently for God to reveal His timetable and His plan. God, however, never gets in a hurry. He has all the time in the world to accomplish His vision for us.

Oswald Chambers, in *My Utmost for His Highest,* says that "God takes us down to the valley to batter us into the shape of that vision. It is in the valley that so many of us give up and faint." He discusses the fact that, while God is busy at work getting us into the shape of the goal He has for us, we are trying to escape from the Sculptor's hand. Rather than trying to batter ourselves into our own goal, we should let the Potter do what He does best. "Then as surely as God is God, you are you, and you will turn out as an exact likeness of the vision."[43]

I am always in awe of Oswald Chamber's wisdom and his understanding of God's character. As I read these familiar words for the "umpteenth" time, I remembered a devotional by Barbara Johnson, one of the Women of Faith writers, in their book, *Boundless Love.* It is a book which several of them autographed for me. In "Diamond Dust," she told about a walk she had taken on a beach on the rugged coast of Maine. As she strolled along the shore, instead of fine sand, she saw stones the size of tennis balls and others as large as basketballs. She said they were all nearly perfectly rounded and smooth. The waves of the wild sea had "transformed the once-jagged rocks into fine objects of beauty."[44]

This is a perfect illustration of God taking us into the valley of Alzheimer's to "batter" us and shape us into something beautiful. Then we, the finished product of God's ongoing process of transformation, will be a great testimony to God's brilliance and skill.

Given the choice, I would not have chosen this process for myself. We all will wish at times that life's seas were not so turbulent and that we could live undisturbed. I have been struck lately about how easily and quickly I can get caught up in the "choppy waters" of life with

---

43   *My Utmost for His Highest:* An Updated Edition in today's Language, edited by James Reimann (Grand Rapids: Discovery House Publishers, 1992), July 6.

44   Barbara Johnson, Boundless Love: Devotions to Celebrate God's Love for You, (Women of Faith Inc., Grand Rapids: Zondervan, 2001), "Diamond Dust", 198.

Alzheimer's. My emotions seem to go from smooth sailing and sunshine to plummeting into dark and stormy waters of a deep sea. The Lord, however, loves us too much to leave us the way we are. Our relationship with Him is a continuing process. So, let's keep on moving forward toward His goal for us. And if we ask Him, like the jeweler, I believe He will use some of His 'diamond dust' to make us into a beautiful jewel. I'm counting on it.

As you are being tossed about in the stormy surf of your life right now, none of this may make any sense to you. You may feel empty and depleted, completely exhausted and hopeless. That's why I'm sharing words of encouragement with you because I've endured many storms on my long journey as an Alzheimer's caregiver. You are welcome to borrow some of my strength, my courage, my hope, my faith, because I care about you.

When you find yourself in a storm, by all means pray that the Lord will remove it. If He doesn't, pray that He will help you to be a witness to those around you in the middle of your storm. We don't want to be guilty of being fair weather Christians. In the midst of a storm, we certainly hope that God will be glorified through us by the way we handle our storm.

I believe that as we keep reflecting Jesus in all that we do for our loved one with Alzheimer's, our progress, our perseverance, and our transformation will be a powerful testimony to a watching world. And we will be beautiful.

My Journal — January 14, 2013

"This morning, a package was delivered to my front door by my mailman because it was too large for my mailbox. It looked like an elephant had jumped on it. He and I laughed because it was stamped with the words, "Damaged but Deliverable." I immediately thought of Barbara Johnson's story in Boundless Love.[45]

45 Ibid, *"Damaged in Transit… But Deliverable."*

After he had left, I thought, "That's how I sometimes feel in this new "season after Alzheimer's." I feel bruised and battered and torn. I want to say "stamp me with the words 'Fragile: Please Handle With Care.' I've been on a long, exhausting journey. I've been pierced with grief and sorrow. I've been crushed, torn, and tattered. I'm still convalescing from a broken heart."

I know this—even though my packaging is torn and ragged, my Father God still recognizes me and accepts me. He reminds me that I will someday be delivered to Him at my home in heaven where I will be perfect. I will have no memory of this difficult time because there will be no more pain, no more sorrow, no more broken hearts." (Lucy)

~ Understanding Through Obedience ~

I believe that God has provided us with this gift because He knows we will have questions as we walk this journey. He also knows that we will not always see things from His perspective.

The truth is, God's ways are beyond understanding. Our friend Job discovered this, and he found himself humbly confessing to God that he had interpreted matters he didn't understand. In Job 42:3, he tells God, "Surely I spoke of things I did not understand, things too wonderful for me to know."

Many times in the last thirteen years, I've been desperate for answers and understanding. So many days, I've longed to sit down with the Lord, face to face, and ask Him, "Why do precious, once busy, productive, even brilliant Christians wander around in Alzheimer's Care facilities, not knowing who or where they are? Aimlessly living out their "golden years" devoid of comforting memories of the past; each day blurring into another—into one long, unknown tomorrow, a tomorrow that will have no memory of the previous day?"

This is how James, my once brilliant, loving, caring, devout Christian husband, lived out his last three years–without the prospect of things ever being different in this life; having no hope for normality except in his new life after death.

Even as I write these word, the Lord is reminding me that I won't ever fully understand any of this. He is Sovereign, and His ways are higher than my ways. In humility, I confess to Him that I believe that He can do all things. Also, even when I don't understand, I must never forget that He is Holy and all powerful and that He is daily unfolding His indisputable plans for me.

C.S. Lewis, in *Mere Christianity*, wrote: "There are a great many things that cannot be understood until after you have gone a certain distance along the Christian road. These are things that are purely practical, though they may not look as if they are. They are directions for dealing with particular crossroads and obstacles on the journey and they do not make sense until a man has reached these places."[46]

Oswald Chambers relates that even when we don't understand, "hang on to the fact that God will ultimately give you clear understanding and will fully justify himself in everything that He has allowed into your life." [47] He also says: "The golden rule for understanding spiritual matters is not intelligence, but obedience."[48]

The Lord tells us in His Word to come to Him for understanding when life becomes too complex and bewildering. He also reminds us that there are some things we don't need to understand; that we only need to trust Him.

I am constantly reminding myself that the Lord has an intimate knowledge and awareness of me, twenty-four hours a day. But I must admit that there have been many days in the past years that I wanted to go into my closet and scream "Help. My world is falling apart. Where are You, Lord?"

My only consolation in those days was the knowledge that Jesus understands my frustration. In His ministry, He made it clear that His followers are not immune to trouble and heartache. His life demonstrated that truth.

The Lord wants us to understand that He knows that this life with Alzheimer's can be pretty ugly, and sometimes our hearts will break.

---

46   *Mere Christianity*, C.S. Lewis, New York, McMillian, 1960, p. 126.
47   Chambers, *My Utmost for His Highest*, Sept 12.
48   Ibid, July 27.

He also wants us to surrender our pain to Him, letting Him heal us. Then, let it go. He understands all of our circumstances. Our purpose-driven Lord never allows trials into our lives unless He has a beautiful purpose for them.

In Romans 8:28, we find the profound promise that we can always cling to and claim: "And we know that in all things God works for the good of those who love him, who have been called according to his purpose." I must have recited that verse hundreds of times in the past thirteen years. This promise is from our Sovereign Lord, who is the ultimate "Promise Keeper." He can turn anything in our lives into a blessing as we love Him and are obedient to His calling.

I believe that the highest privilege we have in this life is to know God and from that knowledge to understand His great love for us. When we remember that God is "love," we will see Him for who He is–not for what He can do for us. Wow. I wonder how many times I have been guilty of thinking of God in that way.

Job said in Job 23:13, "He stands alone, and who will oppose Him? He does whatever he pleases." I believe that in this one verse lies a secret to understanding the mysteries of our circumstances. Our loving Father knows what He is doing. I would not change things, even if I could. Thankfully, I'm wise enough to realize this.

Rather than trying to figure out everything, let's be thankful that we serve a BIG GOD. If we could understand Him, He would be too small to meet our needs.

In July of 1999, when we began our journey with Alzheimer's, James and I made a commitment to trust the promise found in Proverbs 3:5-6, "Trust in the Lord with all your heart and lean not on your own understanding; in all your ways acknowledge him, and he will make your paths straight." Although we didn't always understand, we knew that our faithful Father did.

Even when we don't understand why our loved one is ill with this terrible disease; even when we can't get our minds around the purpose for this tragedy that has disrupted our entire lives, we can rest in God's love. He may not choose to remove our "mountain", but He will give us the strength to climb it, to keep walking, knowing that He is walking with us.

I can assure you from experience, that once you have reached the top of that mountain and have overcome the trials of your journey with Alzheimer's, your life will become a hymn of praise to our loving Lord.

~ Unshakeable Peace ~

"Peace" is a beautiful provision that God our Heavenly Father has promised to His children. We all long for peace: a place to rest our head when our heart is heavy with loss and our bodies and minds are exhausted from the endless tasks and anxiety of caregiving.

Peace, I have discovered, is often elusive because we live in a "broken" world, which was not God's plan when He created it. His solution to the world's "brokenness" is His Son, Jesus, the Prince of Peace.

As caregiver to our loved one with Alzheimer's, we live daily with the uncertainties and frustrations that are part of this terrible disease. That is why it is so important that we unpack God's provision of unshakable peace. He wants us to be the kind of caregivers whose lives and responses to our hardships reflect His peace lived out daily in us. This scripture says it all:

"I've told you all this so that
trusting me, you will be
unshakeable and assured,
deeply at peace. In this
godless world you will
continue to experience
difficulties. But take heart.
I've conquered the world."
John 16:33 (*The Message*).

My Journal – July 29, 2011

"This morning at my Bethel, I'm reading Isaiah 25. This verse particularly spoke to me: "For You have been a defense for the helpless, a shade from the heat; For the breath of the ruthless is like a rain storm against a wall." ~ Isaiah 25:4

I love this devotional about "true peace."

"A contest offered a valuable prize for the best illustration of the concept of peace, and many artists entered. There were renderings of beautiful sunsets over calm seas and hazy scenes of tranquil rivers in lush valleys. But the prize winner's depiction was very different from these tranquil scenes. Painted in black and gray, it depicted the terror of a violent storm. Lightning split the clouds; rain and hail pounded the ground. In the center of the painting was a storm-tossed oak tree. Holding on with all its might to one of the limbs of the tree was a little bird, singing at the top of its lungs. Now, that's true peace."[49]

This devotional went on to say, "ultimate peace is not the absence of storms, but inner peace amidst the storms. And man never finds lasting inner peace until he finds peace with God."[50] (Lucy)

My Journal – December 11, 2009

"Each day, I'm discovering the importance of letting go of the things that weigh me down. Also, I'm determined not to sweat the small stuff. This certainly improves my chances for a peace that allows me to lie down at night and sleep— something that is a scarce commodity in the life of caregivers. It's been ten years since James and I began this journey; ten

---

49   *Peace in the Storm*, Right From the Heart.org.
50   Ibid.

years of watching Alzheimer's slowly but surely rob James of who he once was. This would be a valid reason for me to miss out on God's plan for me to live filled with His promised peace. But I crave this inner peace, and I'm claiming it, regardless of my circumstances.

This is the week of the Singing Christmas Tree at our church. Although I'm trying so hard not to be sad today, my heart is very heavy. I love music, especially Christmas music. I love to sing; I love singing in the Tree. Today I'm wondering if I will ever again be a part of it. Yes, I know that I just wrote about letting go of things that weigh me down, such as memories of the past. I know I must look ahead and stay focused on God's purpose and plans. Only then can I experience peace — something we talk about and sing about so much during the Christmas Season. But just for today, I am grieving for the past.

Normally, by now, I would have my Christmas trees decorated and my entire house, every surface, filled with Christmas items I have collected through the years. The sights and smells of Christmas are some of my favorite things. As I'm sitting here at my "Bethel", writing about "Peace", I'm staring at two small, bare Christmas trees standing on a long, low chest in front of the large living room windows. They have been there for several days. It's as if some giant, icy hand has me in its grip, immobilizing me.

"Father, today I'm being totally honest with You about my needs. I know beyond a doubt that You are in this room with me and that You care about my feelings and my circumstances. This enables me to say with confidence that, with Your help, I can do this. I know that You hold me when I cling to You; when I want to give up. This knowledge of Your faithfulness and love gives me the peace that I so desperately need today. Thank You for always being here, for never leaving me alone, especially when my heart is broken. Will I ever experience the joy of Christmas as I once did? I so much want to. I have so much to be thankful for, I am embarrassed because of my sadness. Forgive me, Father."
(Lucy)

P.S. "My daughter-in-law and my grandson came today and decorated my Christmas trees. This was the best gift they could have given me. Bless Pam and Brett, Father."

My Journal – December 31. 2009

Christmas 2009 has come and gone. The last time I wrote in my journal, I was struggling to take my eyes off myself and to concentrate on Jesus, the reason for the Season. For Christmas, a friend gave me Max Lucado's book, Facing Your Giants. The past few days, when I have some downtime, I'm devouring it. I can relate to so much of what he has written. In one chapter, he writes about "slump guns." He says that "slump guns" fire, not bullets, but sadness; they take, not lives, but smiles; they inflict, not flesh wounds, but faith wounds." He says that "when we're hit, we can't find our rhythm; we can't get out of bed; skies darken and billow; our nights defy sunrise. The "slump gun" mutes the song in our heart; it is the Petri dish for bad decisions."[51]

I think the "enemy" definitely fired his "slump gun" at me this month. This enemy, Satan, knows that, in this strange world of dementia, peace sometimes feels a million miles away. That's where he wants to keep it. God the Father, on the other hand, knowing my desperate need for peace, gives me a breakthrough. There is a moment when I realize that Jesus is standing beside me, protecting me from the enemy's attack, giving me peace in place of my burdens and sadness.

Jesus reminds me that I carry within me the potential for peace wherever I go, whatever I'm facing.

On the eve of a New Year, despite shattered dreams and a deep loneliness in my heart, I'm feeling an unexplainable

---

51   Max Lucado, *Facing Your Giants*, Publisher: MJF Books, 2006.

sense of serenity and peace. Only the indwelling presence of the Holy Spirit could accomplish this. Just now, it's as if God's peace is covering me like a soft, warm blanket. Speaking of blankets, James and I are snuggling together on the sofa, waiting for the bells and whistles and fireworks to usher in the year 2010, and we are content and at peace." (Lucy)

My Journal – January 6, 2010

"Yesterday was an unusually difficult day – one filled with frustrations and challenges. Although I usually try to find a "sitter" for James, I took him with me to the grocery store. I needed to go because our local weather station was predicting unusually cold weather for the next few days, and our fridge and pantry were almost bare. It took me longer than usual to get James up, dressed and fed. Therefore, we got a late start.

At the store, James, who was pushing the grocery cart, got lost from me several times. I had to take him to the bathroom twice, and he wanted to stop and talk to everyone in the very crowded store. When we finally got checked out, I put James in the car, loaded the groceries into the trunk and we started home. By then, it was almost dark.

I stopped at the mailbox around the corner from our house to pick up the mail and to mail two bills that I had stuck in the console of the car. It was then that I realized that the envelopes were missing. When we got home and unloaded the groceries, I settled James into his recliner and then went back out to search the car. By now a fine, cold mist was falling. There was no sign of the bills, and all I could think of was that James had picked them up to look at them while I was loading the groceries and had dropped them when he got out of the car to check on me.

There was no way I could go back to the store to check for myself. I called the store manager to ask that the young sackers and cart boys be on the lookout for the envelopes that were stamped, addressed, and ready to mail. He said he would, and that he would call me if anyone returned them to the store.

By the time I had fed James and gotten him ready for bed, I was exhausted, physically and mentally. After James had gone to sleep, I went to my "Bethel" to pray. I was troubled and discouraged. I asked God for peace and rest. I'm a person who likes to have all the loose ends neatly tied, to know for certain that things are where they should be. After spending some time in prayer, I went to bed.

After several hours of troubled sleep, I woke suddenly, my chest tight with anxiety. I felt like everything was caving in on me, smothering me. I sat up, checked on James and slipped out of bed. I knew that God's Word is filled with promise after promise about His love and faithfulness, and I desperately needed the peace and assurance I knew I would find there. I quickly made my way down the hall to my blue chair, turned on a lamp, wrapped myself in a warm afghan I keep there, and opened my Bible. As I thumbed through the well-worn pages, I stopped each time I saw an underlined or highlighted Scripture. There were so many wonderful words of assurance God had spoken to me in the past and was speaking to me now.

This morning, the sun was coming up as I closed my Bible. I had gone from Genesis to Revelation, reading the marked verses that had given me peace and courage through the years. And I was now at peace.

Incidentally, I found those two bills today, hiding skillfully behind all the mechanisms under the front seats of my car. I believe that the Lord allowed me to misplace those bills because He wanted me to concentrate on the reality of His peace, revealed in His Word. Also, I believe He wants me to share with others what I know and have experienced about His peace that passes all understanding." (Lucy)

I have learned that when life seems to unravel because of my circumstances, I can know that God the Father will step into my circumstances and give me peace. I can know that I carry within me the potential for peace, wherever I go, whatever I am facing. I want my life to "radiate" peace and contentment that comes from my covenant relationship with God. When Jesus said, "My peace I leave with you; my peace I give you," He gave us a gift that comes tied up with the Father's love for us. When we wonder how we can endure the day-in and day-out heartache and frustrations of caring for our loved one, Jesus has a simple answer, "Do not let your heart be troubled." A better interpretation of His words in John 14:27 might be, "Be troubled no longer." This does not mean that we will never experience discouragement or anxiety. It simply means our anxiety will not defeat us or conquer us. It means that Jesus will be with us to give us peace and to bear our anxieties and burdens for us.

When we focus on the Lord instead of our problems, we experience the peace for which He designed us. The Hebrew for "peace" is "Shalom", which means abundance, completeness, fullness, wholeness. These are the very things that describe the life God intended for us before the fall of man in the Garden. When Jesus, the Prince of Peace, rescued mankind from his fallen state, He provided what His Father had planned from the beginning—freedom from worry; life without anxiety, emptiness or hopelessness. Jesus came to bind us back together with God the Father. Because of His great sacrifice for us, we can experience peace even as we deal daily with the "enemy," Alzheimer's.

With the blessed assurance of this unshakable peace from God Himself, let's not complicate our lives with what the world provides – "stuff", status, striving. Instead, let us hold on to this peace that has nothing to do with our circumstances. Even in the reality of our exhaustion, our frustrations, our confusion, our heartache as we recall happier days with our loved one, the peace of God gives us an internal calm, "a peace that passeth understanding."

Just for today, let us claim and enjoy the blessing of God's peace that is:

unexplainable,

indescribable,

illogical,

supernatural, and
unshakable.

P.S. When something tries to rob me of my peace, I will ask myself, "Is this worth the new wrinkles it will cause?"

~ Victory ~

Our Omnipotent God has given us a powerful provision, one we will need on this difficult, often dangerous, and always challenging journey. It's a conditional provision, one we will only receive when we trust Him and wait for Him – it's "Victory." When we fully believe that our battles belong to Him, we get the victory, and He gets the glory. It's a "win/win" situation, my favorite kind.

God's Word portrays hardship and suffering realistically, not as if all problems can be resolved and loose ends always tied up neatly. Life isn't all sweetness and light as we Alzheimer's Caregivers know firsthand. Our battles are real. People in the Bible faced the full gamut of human experience and emotion, from glory and joy to struggles, despair, and ruin. Scripture talks about real people with real challenges, real heartaches, and real suffering. Job, Joseph, Jeremiah, Daniel – these pillars of the faith, and many others who were much loved by God, still experienced profound suffering.

And then, of course, there was Jesus Himself, a Man of Sorrows, well acquainted with pain and suffering. There is one thing that they all share. In the end, they were all victorious.

Our Father wants us to live as if it were impossible to be defeated. When He is involved in our challenges and struggles, our battles are already won because they belong to Him. With Him beside us, the greater the battle, the greater the victory. He gives us the power to overcome any trial or adversity we are facing. Just knowing that my Heavenly Father is fighting my battles for me gives me the courage to be obedient to His marching orders for me. I will be courageous even if those orders involve caring for James twenty-four hours a day, seven days a week.

My Journal – October 21, 2011

"Father, today I'm writing about victory and the importance of standing firm and staying in the fight until, with Your help, we win the victory over every trial. Twelve years ago I discovered that there comes a pivotal time in life when we must face our battles of the heart. Through these years, through my battles, I've learned from time spent with You that my inner strength and courage have a greater purpose than just enabling me to survive day by day. Also, I've discovered that adversity and the resulting pain have developed in me an inner discipline that gives worth and purpose to the very trial that is causing my pain and heartache. Thank You, Father, for revealing this to me. I believe that with Your help, I will never lose the "battle." – I will always, eventually, be victorious." (Lucy)

My battle of the heart began in the long, sleepless nights following James' diagnosis: "Alzheimer's," in July of 1999. It was during those long nights that I claimed an early victory over this faceless, but very real, "Enemy." For the first couple of years, there was very little change in James' behavior. To the casual observer, he was perfectly normal. Even then, however, I realized that victory over this enemy would come only when I surrendered everything to Jesus. "Everything" meant even the inevitable specter of dementia and all the heartache which that entailed. Over a period of time spent on my knees at my Bethel, I gave my fears, my anxieties, my insecurities and inadequacies to Jesus, the greatest Overcomer. As the months and years passed, there were times I wanted to run from this "Enemy" who now had a face—a hateful, leering face. This "Enemy" told me I should surrender when faced with the unthinkable problems of dealing with dementia with its loss of control of bodily functions, loss of logic and reasoning, loss of memory. But as I won victory after victory in my unseen battles of the heart, I learned that, rather than wondering why God would allow this adversity in my life, I could thank Him and trust Him. He honored my trust by revealing to me through time spent in His Word and in prayer, that I was becoming exactly who He had planned for me to be before time began. I learned that facing my worst "Enemy" and my greatest fears with a child-like faith was producing in me something beautiful and lasting – courage.

My Journal – June 28, 2012

"Father, today as I watched the 2012 Olympic Trials, I was reminded that in order to win, I must give all that I have, holding nothing back. I must relentlessly persevere, never wavering until I reach the finish line. Through time spent on my knees, You have taught me that your goal for me is to finish well, to win. My life for the past thirteen years has been a series of trials and tests that I have overcome only with Your help, Father. As I wrote that sentence, I realized that life is much like the Olympic games. It is a test of strength and natural ability honed to perfection by You, Our Master Coach and Trainer. My determination and passion for winning my race comes from You. I will be drawing from Your storehouse of grace, moment by moment, step by step, stride by stride. Thank You that I don't have to run alone; that You are running with me all the way, encouraging me on to victory." (Lucy)

There are always wonderful stories that come from every Olympic Season. There are stories about hardships, conflicts, and miracles. There are stories with intriguing plots of athletes who have overcome tremendous, seemingly impossible hurdles to reach their dreams of competing. Everyone loves a good story, one that ends with ultimate victory, one in which the hero or heroine overcomes and wins a medal.

I don't know about you, but I'm reaching out for the Gold. Jesus is our example of the best story ever written about a battle fought, a race run with patience, and an ultimate victory. His victory, in life and on the Cross, brought glory to His Father in Heaven and eternal life for all who believe in Him and follow Him. I want my story to be all about Jesus as I draw my strength and courage from Him. Daily, I want to become more and more like Him as I care for James and deal with our enemy, Alzheimer's. On the days when I am so tired and discouraged, I will allow Him to fight my battle for me, remembering that the battle is already His. (So is the victory.)

This is a perfect place to share the story of a precious friend, Judy, one of the most courageous women I've ever known. She and her family came and stayed in our home in Houston while she was under treatment for Breast Cancer at M.D. Anderson Hospital. Her doctors at home had done all they could do, and they sent her to Houston where some of the finest Oncologists in the country are located. After a courageous battle on the part of Judy and the doctors, she was sent home to die. Although Judy was heartbroken, she fought hard and well. She purchased small, polished stones and wrote on each one the scripture from 2 Chronicles 20:15. "The battle is not yours, but God's." (I still have mine.) In the months before her death, she touched many lives with her story of faith and determination. Her remaining life, though brief, brought honor and glory to her Heavenly Father. She finished well.

I love the movie, "Rocky Balboa." I watched it with Jesus on TV when it showed recently. I love watching movies with Jesus beside me. If for some reason the movie is offensive, I turn it off. Otherwise, I enjoy watching the stories through His eyes. My favorite line in the movie was Rocky's: "It isn't how many times you're knocked down, but how many times you keep getting up." When Rocky was in the ring for the last time, I was cheering for him, encouraging him, wanting him to finish well, which he did – physically, emotionally, and spiritually. He proved the truth of the scripture read to him by the priest before the fight: "Not by might nor by power but by my Spirit, says the Lord Almighty" (Zechariah 4:6).

My Father wants to hear my story of how, with His grace, I am overcoming. Then He wants me to share my story with everyone, especially you, my fellow caregiver. Remember, to be victorious when our "Enemy", our "Giant," shouts at us, we must shout back. Also remember that the battle is the Lord's, and we never have to lose. With Jesus Christ walking beside us, we will:

✝ Walk like a champion.

✝ Talk like a champion.

✝ Finish like a champion.

When I finally came to the realization that my life in Jesus has eternal significance, I knew that I had gained entrance into that unshakable peace available to me through my faith in Him. I know that someday I will rest eternally from my "battles" at my home in Heaven. And it will have been worth it all when I see Jesus—and James.

"But thanks be to God.
He Gives us the victory though our
Lord, Jesus Christ.
(1 Corinthians 15:57).

~ Wisdom ~

Wisdom is one of the provisions God has packed for our journey, one we can ask for without apology. We know from Scripture that, when Solomon asked God for wisdom rather than riches, honor, or long life,

God granted his request. God knew that I would need this provision of wisdom every day of my journey as James' caregiver. And I know that when I ask for it, God will grant it.

Until July of 1999, James and I were living remarkably blessed and contented lives. We were enjoying our retirement and our little grandsons. We had many friends, and we were active in our church. With James' onset of Alzheimer's, we were faced with the reality of living the rest of his life with an incurable disease. Learning to live with this reality has become my path to wisdom:

Wisdom to follow our Guide,
    to thank God for our trials,
        to search for answers in God's Word,
            to trust that God is always in control,
                to trust God's timing, not my own.

Thankfully, God's wisdom is available every moment of the day. Listen to these instructions: "Trust in the Lord with all your heart and lean not on your own understanding. In all your ways acknowledge Him and He will make your paths straight" (Proverbs 3:5-6). There's that verse again.

The wisdom we need—God's wisdom—is revealed in His Word, by His Spirit and through prayer. Our assignment is to find, follow, and finish the plan as we spend time every day meditating on His Word. When we try to live apart from the counsel of God's wisdom, we suffer disillusionment, fear, doubt, worry, and defeat. Our lives can fall apart when we don't ask God for wisdom in our decision making.

Because God loves us, we have no need to worry about the future. He has a plan, not only for our lives but also for every problem we face. Oswald Chambers said, "All our fretting and worrying is caused by planning without God."[52] Take time today to renew your trust in God and His ability to provide the wisdom you need.

---

52   Oswald Chambers, *My Utmost for His Highest, An Updated Edition in Today's Language*, Edited by James Reimann, (Grand Rapids, Discovery House Publishers, 1992), July 4.

Out of some of my most desperate moments have come my finest moments and my greatest insight into God's character. I have learned that when I come to the Lord in a simple act of worship, I am providing Him a way to permeate my heart with His wisdom. In Eugene Peterson's *The Message*, 1 Kings 4:29 reads, "God gave Solomon wisdom—the deepest understanding and the largest of hearts. There was nothing beyond him, nothing he couldn't handle."

That's the kind of wisdom I prayed for as James' logic and reasoning became increasingly impaired. Until this time, James and I had always made every decision together. Now I was faced with the stark realization that this was becoming less and less an option.

One of the areas in which I needed divine wisdom had to do with our automobiles—whether to keep or to trade. I would discuss things with James, the all-time expert in such matters, but ultimately the decision was left to me. So I prayed earnestly for wisdom and, as usual, God showed up. He sent a wonderful "angel" in the form a fleet manager for a car dealership. From the time we met him in 2000, he took care of our car needs, handling all the details of repairs, trading, buying, and then leasing until James' death in 2012. In 2009, he not only found the car I had decided on, he picked it up, went to our doctor's office for the form needed for handicap license plates, went by the courthouse to pick up the plates, drove into our driveway and put the plates on for us. God never does anything halfway. (Neither did our automobile angel).

Probably my most profound need for God's wisdom was the need to know when I could no longer leave James alone. The Bible is filled with assurances of God's faithfulness in giving us wisdom. My favorite is found in James 1:5, "If any of you lacks wisdom, he should ask God, who gives generously to all without finding fault, and it will be given to him." One day when I was praying, God's spirit directed me to this verse. When I read it with fresh eyes, I knew that the "you" meant me. And so I asked with all the faith in me, believing every word of this promise.

My Journal – December 11, 2007

The Night of the Flood

"As James' logic and reasoning became more and more impaired by the progression of his Alzheimer's, I began to ask God daily for divine wisdom in the area of leaving him at home alone.

In December of 2007, I was still leaving James alone for short periods while I attended various church activities and functions. Our church is so close I can see it from my front door. Singing in the choir at our church is one of my greatest joys. The Singing Christmas Tree was one of the highlights of the year, and in 2007, as usual, I was eagerly involved. There were five performances, with two on Saturday, a matinée and an evening performance. Missing even one of them was out of the question for me, and I was comfortable leaving James for an hour or two. I was planning to take him to the Sunday evening performance, and my son would be with him Thursday, Friday, and Saturday nights. On Saturday, after the matinée, I decided to go home and take a brief afternoon rest before the evening performance. Climbing into and standing in the "tree" for over an hour can be very tiring, although, for a seventy-three-year-old. I can climb with the best of them.

I had just stretched out in my recliner in the den when James came into the room from our bedroom down the hall. He looked distraught, and he tugged on my arm as he said, "I need a little help here." The Understatement of the Year. I hurried down the hall and through our bedroom. When I reached the bathroom, I was met by a "rushing river" caused by an overflowing commode in our "potty" room. I walked through inch deep water to turn off the water at the wall, something James had taught me to do fifty years before. Then I started grabbing every towel and bath rug I could find to stop the water before it flowed into our bedroom. Just a few months before, I had the carpet in our bedroom replaced with beautiful wood floors. I took blankets and throws off our bed and chairs to put at the bathroom door and along the walls just inside our bedroom.

All this time James was standing by helplessly, saying, "I didn't do this. I didn't cause this." I was probably rather hysterical at this point, but when I realized how traumatized he was, I tried to reassure him and calm him; I stopped long enough to hug him and to get him settled in his recliner in our bedroom.

When I had soaked up all the visible (thankfully, relatively clear) water, I called a friend's cell phone to let the choir director know I would not be in the tree that night. As I looked at all the wet towels, blankets, rugs, and throws that now filled our large spa bathtub, I had a brief "praise and thanksgiving service." I thanked God that I was at home when this occurred. I shuddered to think what would have happened had I not been there. It was one of those moments when you know, without a doubt, that God has protected you from what would have been a total disaster—a totally flooded house.

There is a Scripture, Proverbs 2:8, which perfectly describes God's personal involvement in the lives of His children. It reads, "For He guards the course of the just and protects the way of his faithful ones."

With James safely settled in his recliner, I began to fill large plastic garbage bags with wet towels, rugs, and blankets. Do you know how heavy wet towels, rugs and blankets are? I found out. But God, as usual, showed up with the extra strength and stamina I needed. He also protected my back from injury. Through all of this, James slept in his recliner.

Before the night was over, I had filled and carried ten large garbage bags to the laundry room. The washer and dryer had a very busy night. As did I. I mopped and sterilized and mopped and sterilized some more, almost asphyxiating myself with Clorox bleach. (Did I mention I'm a registered nurse, obsessed with "sterile techniques?) By eleven o'clock, I had done all I could do. I left a message for a company that specializes in Macrobiotics treatment of water damaged areas. Then I went to bed.

I can assure you, no one had to rock me to sleep. My last thought that night, "the night of the flood," as I will always refer to it in the future, was to thank my Heavenly Father. I thanked Him for showing me, as only He can, that I could never again leave James at home alone. And I haven't. This was His answer to my daily prayer for wisdom.

My life changed dramatically after that night. James and I were now officially "Homebound." More importantly, my faith was greatly strengthened through this experience. I had learned even more about God's character:

✝ *He always provides peace and joy when we allow Him into our circumstances.*

✝ *Nothing can touch His children apart from His permissive will.*

✝ *His wisdom and strength are available to me twenty-four hours a day, every day, just when I need them. (Lucy)*

My Journal – December 18, 2008

"Attention: Little Man Lost": December 13, 2008

"After the "flood" last December, I continued to faithfully consult God and seek His wisdom concerning James' safety. I never left him at home alone after that day, a day when God answered my prayer for His wisdom. Now, every day I pray for wisdom for the next step of our journey.

There is a small but wonderful mall near our home. I shop there often because it does not require freeway driving; it is only five or six minutes from our home and I can park in front of each shop or business. My nail salon is there, and James looks forward to going with me because everyone there knows and loves him. He loves them, too, as he does everyone. He always asks every woman there if they have always been "that pretty" and tells the salon owner that he is "too wonderful to be real." Sometimes he sits there on a couch near the door while I shop for a few minutes next door at Bath and Body Works.

Last week, on December 13, 2008, after our usual rounds of the salon and several stores, I decided to drive further down the mall to look for a "Little Einstein" book and game I had seen earlier in a store there. I wanted them for a Christmas gift for our four-year-old grandson. James was very tired by then, and he begged to stay in the car while I ran into the store. Because the weather was cool, and because I found a parking place in front of the store, I agreed. I rolled the front windows down a few inches, locked the doors, and gave James firm instructions to remain in the car. After promising to be gone only fifteen minutes, I hurried into the store. I quickly found the book and game, paid for them and was back to the car in exactly fifteen minutes.

I was at the car before I realized that James was gone. With my heart pounding and feeling faint with fear, I ran back into the store I had just left, thinking that maybe he had gone to the restroom there, and I had missed him. No James. After having him paged and giving instructions to keep him there if he appeared, I ran into the stores on either side, looked for him and had him paged. Still no James. I knew he was not able to walk very far. By then, I was past frantic. I started praying and running through the parking lot, looking into cars and asking everyone I met if they had seen him.

Just as I started walking further down the long sidewalk, thinking he couldn't possibly have walked that far, my cell phone rang. It was my daughter-in-law, Pam, calling to say that James was with her, further down the mall. James had walked down past the James Avery store where, miraculously, a friend from our church was working part-

time. She recognized James and called my daughter-in-law at the church where she is the Children's Minister. The friend kept James with her until Pam arrived a few minutes later and put James into her car to wait for me.

I was so relieved and happy to see James, and he was happy to see me. He said, "I couldn't find you. I thought you were lost." We hugged and cried. I felt like a mother whose little boy was lost, who didn't know if she would ever see him again. I realized then that James is my "little man," my full-time responsibility.

Never again would I leave James alone in a car or anywhere. I thanked God over and over again for miraculously keeping him safe. I knew that once again, my faithful Father in Heaven had answered another of my prayers for wisdom."
(Lucy)

My Journal – August 31, 2009

Innocence Lost

"August 15, 2009, will forever be engraved in my mind as one of the most traumatic days of my life. I call it the "day we lost our innocence." Even now, two weeks later, I can scarcely bear to think about it.

It was a Saturday, and our grandsons had come for the weekend. Because it had been a rainy week, I had not been grocery shopping, and I needed several things. We went to our local supermarket. Yes, it was the infamous store where several months before I had been a witness to a violent robbery of the bank located in the store.

James liked going to this store with me because there is a snack area with tables, near the door we enter and by the restrooms. By the time we walk from the car into the store, James is exhausted and anxious to sit down at one of the tables. Many of the store employees know James because we shop there every week and because he is so friendly. After getting him a cookie and assuring him that I would check on him often, I would begin shopping. At the end of each aisle, I always checked on him and waved and he would wave back.

On this day, I was halfway through the second aisle when I looked up to see James coming toward me. I said, "Do you want to walk with me and push the cart for awhile?" Then I realized we were not alone. A young police officer and another man, who I learned later was one of the store managers, had followed James into the aisle, which thankfully was empty except for us. The police officer walked up to James and said, "Sir, I need to talk to you." I immediately said, "You need to talk to me. My husband has Alzheimer's and does not communicate well. What's wrong?" The officer said, "Your husband has badly frightened and traumatized a little girl, and her parents are very upset."

I was at that point not believing what I was hearing. I asked if James had touched or hurt the little girl in any way. He didn't answer me. I began explaining that James would never hurt anyone, especially a child. I told him that James had most likely asked the little girl if she had "always been that pretty."

James, by then, was looking pale and very confused. He kept saying, "Am I in trouble? Did I do something wrong?" This from a man who, to my knowledge, had never done or said anything to hurt anyone. I assured him that he had done nothing wrong. Then I wasted no time telling the young officer this. I explained that James was the most righteous man I'd ever known; that he was a deacon in our large church down the street; that we had lived in Pasadena for forty years and had raised our children there; that he had *retired from Shell Oil Company, where he was an executive; that we had hundreds of friends in the area.*

I looked at the name on the officer's badge and realized his mother was a teacher in the school district where our son had taught and coached. I told him this and suggested that our son had probably coached him, (which he had).

I was trying to be calm and Christ-like as I'm saying all this, but I was very upset. I had led a very sheltered life, never having so much as a traffic ticket. Then, after all that I had said, the young officer walked right up to James, got right in his face and asked, "Sir, are you a registered sex offender?" At first I was so stunned, I couldn't speak. Then I stepped between my sweet James and this young, rude police officer.

Right in his face I said, "I can't believe you just asked that. Did you not hear one word I said?" If I was upset before, I was traumatized at this point and furious. I felt like a mother lion must feel when she thinks her cub is in danger. I was shaking all over. I couldn't remember being really angry ever before in my life. I was "fighting mad." I demanded that we be allowed to talk to the parents and the little girl. I wanted them to see that this sweet, godly, eighty-three-year-old man was ill and that he would never have hurt her—or anyone. I wanted them to see that he was probably much more traumatized than she. The officer said we could not talk to them and the store manager said they had left the store.

The officer then said to me, "You can't bring him back to this store again." Whoa! A red flag immediately went up in my mind. I said, "Do you mean to tell me that all handicapped, mentally-challenged people are banned from this store? And what happened to the Alzheimer's / Dementia Sensitivity training that I thought was a part of the Police Academy Training?" (I wanted to ask him, "were you absent that day?")

I was still too much in shock to express everything I was feeling. By then I had taken James' hand and was trying to decide whether to turn my grocery cart upside down, dumping everything on the floor and then leaving the store. I would have never done anything like that, but it made me feel better just to imagine it.

While I am visualizing this, the young officer was joined by a young woman officer. He then asked James' age and birthday, which I graciously gave. Then they left. And I did the most Christ-like thing I could think of doing. I put my arm around James, asked him to be quiet and to stay very close to me, and we finished our shopping.

James was pale and very quiet during all this. I tried to act as normal as possible even though I was sick inside. As we checked out, I smiled and talked to the checkers and sackers who all knew us. When we were finally in the car, leaving the parking lot, James said, with tears in his eyes. "Let's don't ever come here again." I was surprised at his clarity of mind at that point, and I promised him we would never go there again. And we didn't.

Before the day was over, James had forgotten all that had happened, but I could not. This wound I had received was still too open and raw. I wanted someone else to hurt, those who had hurt us, but God reminded me that this was His job, not mine. My job, He reminded me, was to roll all this hurt and anger over on Him.

The next morning as I drove the short distance to our church to teach my Sunday Bible Study class, God said, "Let it go, Lucy." And I did. Monday morning I had a long, very healing phone conversation with the embarrassed store manager who, according to him, had experienced a miserable weekend. He seemed relieved to be able to express his regrets and to ask for my forgiveness. He said he didn't realize who James was until he saw us together there in the aisle. We discussed the importance of being sensitive to Alzheimer's sufferers and their families. I told him that because I was a Christian, I would not file discrimination charges against the store, something I had been advised by an elder law attorney that I should do. The manager seemed relieved, and he thanked me and again expressed his regrets.

After I had hung up the phone, I thanked God for peace and closure and for the graphic answer to my prayers for wisdom. I knew now that I could never again leave James alone, even when I was nearby in the same store. From then on he would walk at my side wherever we were. I could sense that the "winds of change" were again blowing in what was once our safe, uncomplicated, secure world. I wondered what tomorrow and all the days and months ahead would bring, but I didn't need to wonder who would be walking with us. I knew. It would always be our faithful, loving Guide, our Father God." (Lucy)

Decision Making: 101

In February 2010, I found myself at the "end of my rope," but once again at the beginning of God's wisdom. James and I had been homebound the past two years. God had given me the wisdom I needed to make some serious decisions about James' safety and welfare during the years 2008 and 2009. Christmas Eve 2009, brought a new challenge and a new danger. Sometime after midnight I was suddenly awakened when the alarm system on our front door said, "Front door open." I looked over and realized that James was not in bed. I raced to the front door that was standing open. Then I saw James, barefoot, and in his underwear, standing at the end of our front sidewalk. It was very cold, and I, too, was barefoot and robeless. I ran to James and said, "Honey, what are you doing out here? It's cold. Come inside." He said, "No, I have to go." When I asked him where he was going, he pointed to the intersection at the end of our street and said, "I'm going home." By then, I had him headed back toward the front door, explaining that he was home, that we had lived there for ten years. Still protesting that he wasn't home, he allowed me to lead him back into the house and back to bed. He was very cold, and I added an extra blanket to his cold feet and legs. As I got into bed and held him close, I thanked God for His protection and love. I also thanked Him for giving me the wisdom to install a Home Security System the past Spring. Without its warning alarm, James might have been hopelessly lost on that cold December night. At bedtime, I had been very tired after having friends and family over for dinner before the Christmas Eve Candlelight service at our church. Exhausted as I was, I might not have waked up until morning.

Now, a few weeks later, I am faced with another huge decision concerning James' safety. The further James and I go on this journey, the more decisions I must make. I've always had difficulty making decisions, but I'm very good at making lists—lists with columns with the headings: "pros" and "cons." That's not necessarily a bad thing, but I've learned that the wisest thing to do is to consult the One who already has all the answers, my Father in Heaven. On this journey with Alzheimer's, I've learned some valuable lessons about making God-sized decisions. I call this "Decision Making: 101."

- Identify the problem. (God already has.)

- Talk to the Lord about it. (He already knows about it.)

- Listen for the answer. (He has the answer and He wants you to know it.)

- Stand still until you receive His answer. (As long as you're still, you won't get in His way.) Exodus 14:14: "The Lord will fight for you; you need only to be still."

- Wait until you see the Lord at work, and then trust Him and follow Him. (He will make the path straight and clear, removing all obstacles. The key word here is "trust.") Psalm 62:6, Proverbs 3:6

- When you don't have a plan, ask God for His. (Remember, He knows the plans He has for you.) Jeremiah 29:11

- Ultimately, always choose what you will be satisfied with in the future. (God's wisdom makes this possible.)

Many of my decisions on this journey have been a tug-of-war between realism and optimism. As James' caregiver, I've tried through the years to make decisions I arrived at after much prayer, because I always wanted to do what was best for James. I decided after the diagnosis, "Alzheimer's," that there were no simple rules for this journey, only the need to be honest and flexible. I made a commitment that I would submit to God's will and trust that He was powerful enough and wise enough to monitor our circumstances. It was the wisest decision I could have made. Had it not been for the wisdom and insight that God has given me through the past eleven years, I would have been tempted to "throw in the towel." Instead, I've learned to live in awesome reverence for God, resulting in a wisdom that is beyond human understanding.

"Thank You, Father, for empowering me to walk with confidence and wisdom through all the days of this journey, the good days and the difficult ones. Please help me to wait for your wisdom and instructions for the next part of this journey. Help me to be obedient, however difficult the next miles may be. And always keep James safe when I can't be with him. Amen."

With the wisdom that God gave me, I was able to make the painful, but wise decision to sell our home and to move with James to a Brookdale Senior Living Community with Assisted Living and a wonderful Memory Care Program. I discussed this at length elsewhere in the book.

~ Worship Opportunities ~

The Bible tells us that we were created by God to praise Him and to worship Him. For the first forty-three years of our marriage, James and I worshiped and served God together each Sunday in our church. After the year 2000, James could no longer serve as he had always done, but he loved attending church and worshiping God.

Even as his Alzheimer's advanced, he could sing most of the old familiar hymns and many of the newer praise songs. He could find Scripture passages in his Bible, and he always said "Amen" at the appropriate times. It was during this time that I began to realize that the Spirit of God within us never gets dementia. If I had ever needed proof that God's Spirit dwells within us, it was confirmed by James' ability to worship and praise God as he had always done. Until 2008, with the help of some of the deacons and our son David, James was able to sit in the church service while I sang in the choir at our church.

You may not have grown up attending church. Perhaps you have never been a part of worship and praise in a church setting. Even so, God has wisely packed this provision for us on our journey with Alzheimer's. He knows that when we come to Him in our times of desperation, and He meets us in that moment of need, we will come away transformed. As we experience His faithfulness, we will find ourselves exalting Him with our thoughts, attitudes and actions wherever we are. That's what worship is.

Do you ever long to leave all the drudgery, the sickness, and sadness behind for just a little while? Would you like a break sometime to just get away from it all, to go to a place where you can just leave it all behind? That is what worship does. Hebrews 4:15-16 tells us, "Let us then approach the throne of grace with confidence so that we may receive mercy and grace to help us in our time of need."

In the Bible, the word "worship" means to bow in humble respect to a superior being. When Jesus came, He taught that more important than our physical posture was the attitude and posture of our heart. Later, in Mark 7, Jesus teaches that it is useless to honor God with our lips (or our posture) while our hearts are far from Him. If our heart does not "kneel," we have failed to worship the Lord.

Since the year 2000, I have been teaching an 8:30 A.M. Bible Study class of Senior Single Adults at our church, the church I can see from our front door. By the year 2008, I was no longer able to take James to church on Sunday morning. Our son Matt would care for his Dad while I went to teach my class. I returned home by 9:45 A.M. so that he could then attend church. At home, I would watch a sermon on television. There I had my own special worship time with God while James slept down the hall in our bedroom.

ᏣᎠ

My Journal – September 10, 2009

"Shortly after we moved into our "miracle house" on Rainbow Bend in November of 1999, I discovered a "sanctuary" in our living room. Most people don't live in their living room, much less worship there. This has been, for the past

ten years, my "Bethel." It is the place I hurry to every morning, usually before dawn. I can scarcely wait to get down the long hall from our bedroom to my blue chair, my Bethel. Here I spend time on my knees talking to and listening to my Father. Even though I may have been talking to Him all through the night, I treasure this special time and place where He meets me every morning. I read several of the Psalms, which I pray back to Him, and usually some verses from Paul's letters to the early churches. I also read the devotional for the day from Oswald Chamber's wonderful My Utmost for His Highest, looking up the scripture for that date. So many times the thoughts and scripture passages of the day are exactly what I need for that moment.

I'm writing these words after a restless night. James was up several times, disoriented as usual. He's always restless even when asleep. I'm like a mother of a small child, aware of every movement and every sound he makes during the night. He always needs to be touching me, holding my hand, being reassured that I am there. He never feels safe. I try to think how frightening it would be to not know who you are or where you are, especially in the dark of night. The scripture for the day, September 10, in My Utmost for His Highest, is John 1:48, "When you were under the fig-tree, I saw you." The lesson is "Worshiping in Everyday Occasions." Oswald Chambers says that "a private relationship of worshiping God is the greatest essential element of spiritual fitness." He stresses the importance of "worshiping in everyday occasions in our home." He concludes the day's devotional with the truth that "God's training ground is the hidden, personal worshiping life of the saint."

As I read the words about worshiping in our home, I remember a day several weeks ago that perfectly illustrates this thought. James and I were sitting in our living room watching a storm approaching from the north. We haven't had much rain this summer, and none for several weeks. I was excited by the prospect of our yard being watered by our Heavenly Father rather than by me. There are four large floor-to-ceiling windows in the room, and we could watch the dark clouds coming nearer, accompanied by rumbling thunder, wind and lightning flashes. I love storms as long as I'm not out in them. I always feel so close to God, the Creator, as he unleashes His power. Psalm 104: 1, 3 says, "Praise the Lord, my soul. He makes the clouds his chariot and rides on the wings of the wind."

As the rain began to fall in torrents, washing the windows with the help of the strong wind, I expressed my gratitude and praise to God. I looked at James, sitting on the couch opposite the windows and I said, "Honey, God is so good. Aren't we blessed with this rain?" He raised his hands in the air, closed his eyes, and said, "Thank You, Lord. Thank You for the rain." Then he got down on his knees (a small miracle), and with hands still raised, he looked toward heaven and thanked God again. My eyes filled with tears, just as they are doing now as I write. I felt at that moment that we should take off our shoes because we were truly on "holy ground." As my heart almost burst with joy from what I was experiencing, I realized that this was pure, unadulterated, and true worship. There was no church building, no worship center, no order of worship, no organ music, no choir, no sermon from the pulpit, no invitation, no benediction. There were only the two of us and Jehovah God in our living room on an ordinary day made extraordinary by this unforgettable time of worship. Something extraordinarily sacred was taking place, and I knew we were witnessing a glimpse of Heaven on earth.

1 Chronicles 16:29b reads, "Worship the Lord in the splendor of his holiness." That is exactly what we were doing on that stormy day. I made a promise that day to never again feel sorry for myself because I could no longer be at church for every worship service, every event, every meeting, or because I could no longer be singing in the choir every Sunday as I had done for years. As much as I miss those things, I have found my sanctuary, not just in my blue-chair-Bethel in my living room, but in my heart. As the song says, "With thanksgiving, I'll be a living Sanctuary for Thee." (Lucy)

As I'm spending more and more time alone with God, my private worship time with Him takes my eyes off my problems and lifts them to Him, our Burden Bearer. *Romans 12:1, The Message* reads, "Take your everyday, ordinary life—Your sleeping, eating, going-to-work, and walking around life and place it before God as an offering." My ordinary, everyday life? The drudgery, the unthinkable tasks, the despair, the exhaustion? Can I offer these to Holy God? Yes. I believe that is exactly what Paul meant when he was inspired to write those words. I'm also learning that when I receive a blessing from God, I can give it back to Him as a love offering in an intentional act of praise and thanksgiving.

I'm discovering that when I focus my heart and mind on God, wherever I am, He is exalted, and my burdens are lighter. Helen Lemmel wrote a song in 1922 that we sang in college in the 1950s. Sometimes, I find myself singing the words in my times of worship,: "Turn your eyes upon Jesus. Look full in His wonderful face. And the things of earth will grow strangely dim in the light of His glory and grace." [Pubic domain]

Adrian Rogers, in one of his televised sermons, stated that "the Heavens always declare the glory of God, but sometimes we forget to look up."

As we face each day with its challenges, let us turn our eyes on Jesus. Let us remember to look up and see God revealed in His awesome creation, and let us worship Him in His holiness. I know from experience how comforting and strengthening that personal, intimate worship time can be.

I love thinking about and writing about worship. Worship is part of my DNA. Not only does worshiping God bring peace and joy and fulfillment into our lives, but it also has some great physical benefits. Max Lucado, in *Grace for the Moment,"* one of my favorite daily devotional books, describes these benefits. He says that when we worship God and seek His face, He, in turn, will change our face. "By his fingers, wrinkles of worry are rubbed away. He relaxes clenched jaws and soothes furrowed brows. His touch can remove the bags of exhaustion from beneath the eyes and turn tears of despair into tears of peace." [53]

---

53   July 3, page 208.

Wow. Our "Bethel" can become our private spa when we worship God and seek His face. I don't know about you, but I'm heading there now.

Of course, I can never write about worship without writing about music. Music-initiated worship is the first worship I experienced as a small child. One of my earliest memories is sitting on the front row of our church with other five and six-year-olds. We were singing *Jesus Loves The Little Children of the World*, and I remember being so moved by my love for the children in Africa, I was singing with all my heart. Our minister stepped off the platform, picked me up and set me down on the stage where I finished "belting out" the words, "Jesus loves the little children. All the children of the world." Not only was I worshiping God that day, I was surrendering my heart to missions.

The wonderful hymns of my childhood helped to open my heart to God. Then came the wonderful praise and worship choruses that not only talk about God but allow us to sing back to Him our praise and worship for all of His attributes. They tell the old, old story in a fresh, new, relevant way. Some of my favorites: *Blessings*, sung at James' funeral and *When the Hurt and the Healer Collide*, my inspiration for the chapter about God's provisions for our journey with Alzheimer's. I also love *Jesus, Be The Center of It All*, which inspires me to rededicate my life to Jesus every time I hear it. Great hymns of the faith like *Great is Thy Faithfulness, It is Well With My Soul, and Blessed Assurance* give me words and melodies that sing in my heart and help me to express my praise when my heart is too heavy and too bruised to sing.

Our youngest son, a worship pastor with a doctorate in worship studies, could sing before he could talk. I think that may have come from hearing me sing to him before he was born. For the three months before his birth at the end of December, I had been rehearsing music for our annual Christmas cantata. I sang to a tape of the music every day during the months of October, November, and December, learning the words and music.

All three of our sons were exposed to music from birth. Nothing was more touching than watching their sweet mouths struggling to sing the words, "Jesus loves me, this I know, for the Bible tells me so."

I read somewhere that Karl Barth, the great theologian, when asked if he could condense all of the theology he had ever written into one sentence, said "Yes I can. Jesus loves me this I know for the Bible tell me so."

Just think, 'our babies' minds and hearts have been saturated with the truth that Jesus loves them. All this through the words and music of a simple, yet profound song.

I agree with Martin Luther, who once said, "Next to the Word of God, music deserves the highest praise. The gift of language, combined with the gift of song, was given to man that he should proclaim the Word of God through music."[54]

The Minister of Music at our church, once wrote in his column in our church publication, "We should not come to a worship service to see what we can get out of it, but rather for one purpose, to give our praise to God."

Music may not be your "thing." Praise and worship may be something of a new or foreign concept to you. But remember this: worship is the purpose for which we were created. When I think of God's attributes and of all the ways that He has blessed me, worshiping Him comes naturally for me.

For the rest of my life here on earth, I want my worship to be more than just a song. I want to worship God, not just with words but with my entire life—with my talents, my creativity. I want my very life, even as a caregiver, to be an act of worship. I will remember: "Worship matters."

I have experienced God and have lived long enough in His presence that whatever I'm doing, even the menial tasks involved with caring for James, has become an act of worship. I pray that you, too, will realize this as you care for your loved one.

~ Extraordinary Living ~

God our Heavenly Father is extraordinary, and it has been His plan from the beginning that His children would experience extraordi-

---

54   Source Unknown

nary living. Synonyms for extraordinary are: remarkable, exceptional, astonishing, sensational, incredible, unbelievable, phenomenal.

God has packed this provision for us, knowing that we are facing many trials and crises on our journey. Thankfully, our pain and heartache cannot keep us from the extraordinary life that He offers, life only He can give. Extraordinary living is not something we do for ourselves. God does it for us. How extraordinary.

Let's look at Romans 12:1,. "So here's what I want you to do, God helping you: Take your everyday, ordinary life—your sleeping, eating, going-to-work, and walking–around life and place it before God as an offering. Embracing what God does for you is the best thing you can do for him" (The Message).

That verse tells me to take everything in my life of caregiving— the worry, the fear, the drudgery, the heartache—and give them to God as an offering, as an act of worship. This is the process by which I accept the extraordinary life God has planned for me. I don't know about you, but I want it all. I don't want to be satisfied with anything less than His extraordinary best for me.

In one of my favorite movies, "Mr. Magorium's Emporium," Mr. Magorium says, "Life is an occasion. Rise to it." God calls us, just ordinary caregivers, from our difficult, lonely, drudgery-filled, exhausting, frustrating lives to His extraordinary living.

Ephesians 1:14 (The Message) tells us, "this signet from God is the first installment on what's coming, a reminder that we'll get everything God has planned for us, a praising and glorious life." What an extraordinary promise.

Oswald Chambers says that you should live "in constant wonder, because you don't know what God is going to do next." Until I read this on January 2 in My Utmost for His Highest, I thought I was unique in my "faith process" about this very thing. As far back as I can remember, I've always approached life with the attitude, "Lord, I can't wait to see what You're going to do next in my life." So, I was excited when I read Eugene Peterson's paraphrase of Romans 8:15, The Message: "This resurrection life you received from God is not a timid, grave–tending life. It's adventurously expectant, greeting God with a childlike "What's next, Papa?"

I believe that my loving, thoughtful Abba Father knew I would need this deeply ingrained faith in Him as I face the daily unknowns of life with Alzheimer's. Being certain of God helps me to deal with the daily uncertainties of this journey.

✂

My Journal – April 13, 2012

Early this morning, my phone rang. It was the Manager at Clare Bridge, the Memory Care Facility at the Hampton. He said that something was wrong with James. He didn't want to get up; he seemed depressed. After he had been persuaded to let himself be dressed, he refused to leave his recliner to go to breakfast. All of this was totally out of character for James, who is normally easy-going and happy.

I dressed quickly and made the short, thirty-second trip from the house we had built the previous summer. On the way I was praying, not knowing what to expect, but believing that God knew exactly what was happening. I know that, if he lives long enough, James may slip into that last stage of Alzheimer's—the stage where he won't be able to recognize me or to function on his own. I have learned in these thirteen years to surrender everything to God, knowing, even in my uncertainty, that He is sufficient and gracious and loving. When I arrived at Clare Bridge and made my way down the hall to James' room, I knew my Father was walking with me. James was slumped down in his recliner, dressed and combed, but sleeping. He looked so precious, but fragile, as I went to him, bending to kiss him gently, greeting him tenderly. When he opened his eyes, I held my breath until he grinned and said, "You're my wife." Tears of joy and relief blinded me for a moment. Then, with a little teasing and prodding, I got him up with the promise that we were going to breakfast together in "our beautiful dining room." As he ate, with a little help from me, I thanked God and rejoiced that, even in the uncertainties of life, He is faithful. (Lucy)

That day I was reminded again that, when I am in the right relationship with God, my days and moments will be filled with "spontaneous, alert expectancy." For the rest of this journey, I will intentionally remain abandoned to God, experiencing the extraordinary living that He has planned for me.

God has revealed this truth to me: extraordinary living is not doing extraordinary things but doing simple, loving things for others in an extraordinary way, with extraordinary love. This kind of servanthood and love allows us to lovingly and patiently change those soiled Depends. To clean up endless puddles. To wade through the unmentionable "messes" in the day of a caregiver. Dementia will either defeat us or make us into beautiful vessels of servanthood for God.

I've come to believe that the worst part of having dementia must be the feeling of being a burden, of being unwanted, of loss of worth and purpose. I see the terrible loneliness in some of those I see daily as I visit my husband. Although the Care Associates and staff at *Clare Bridge* are wonderful and loving, these residents long to be wanted and valued by the significant people in their lives—their children and grandchildren, their spouses, their friends, and former neighbors, people from their church. I am so fortunate that I live less than a minute away from my husband James. I visit him several times every day, and while I'm there, I "love on" those who have few visitors. I will continue as long as possible to help dispel the feeling of abandonment felt by these, believing that God has called me to this ministry, a ministry to share His extraordinary love.

There are so many problems in our fallen world that it's easy to feel as if one person's efforts can't do much to fix them. But God calls every believer to help solve the world's problems, and one ordinary person's life can make an extraordinary impact on their world, where they live.

We can make the world a better place through our life as caregivers. When we rely on God to help us impact our world, His power will start to work through us in our neighborhood, our workplace, our doctor's office, our grocery store, our pharmacy, our bank, our church, and everywhere else we go. We have the extraordinary potential to impact the world around us with our peace and serenity, our love and compassion, our joy and friendliness – and our courage.

Every morning when we open our eyes, we need to realize that the day is a gift, loaded with special things to experience and special opportunities to make a difference in our world and to our loved ones. Every day, every moment, every breath is a beautiful, extraordinary gift given to us by God, who puts the "extra" into the ordinary. So today, live courageously, realizing that yours is a "High Calling" issued by the Commander of the Angel Armies.

~ Yearning for More of God ~

"He said to me: 'It is done, I am the Alpha and the Omega, the
Beginning and the End. To him who is thirsty I will give
to drink without cost from the spring of the water of life'"
(Revelation 21:6).

The Christian walk is not simply about giving up our self-focused desires. It's giving up our right to ourselves in order to be Christ-focused, receiving all that God has planned for us. When our Father packed into our hearts this provision of yearning, thirsting, hungering, and longing to experience more of Him, He knew that the more our hearts yearned for Him, the more diligently we would follow Him. I am so grateful that He knew that out of my desperate needs as James' caregiver would come a newfound intimacy with Him. He knew I would find joy and peace welling up, filling my weary heart every time I felt depleted.

I grew up with the concept that every person is born with a God-shaped, empty place in his heart. As a college student and young adult, I heard friends and acquaintances asking, "What is life all about?" It seemed that everyone my age was searching desperately for answers and for meaning in their lives. As a believer and follower of Jesus, I was blessed to have the answer: Jesus Christ. He is the answer. I knew that the emptiness my friends were experiencing was a yearning and a thirst for a Living God to give purpose to their lives, and I shared my faith with them.

Psalm 42:1-2 states it beautifully: "As the deer pants for streams of water, so my soul pants for you, O God. My soul thirsts for God, for the living God. When can I go and meet with God?" That question, asked from the heart of the psalmist, is the constant prayer of my heart. I know that only God can meet my needs as I walk this "uncharted" path of caregiving.

The Lord will never disappoint us when we yearn for and seek His will. We may at times feel disappointed or let down when the things we yearn for and pray for are not in His plans for us. We must remember, however, that He wants only the best for His children. We can't even imagine the good things that God has in store for each of us. Proverbs 10:24 tells us that "what the righteous desire will be granted." Remember, God always keeps His promises. Some things we can be sure of:

We are not walking our journey alone.

We have Someone bigger and wiser than ourselves on which to lean.

We have a God who is our Burden-bearer and our strength when we're exhausted.

We have a Shelter and safe haven in the storms.

We have a loving Companion when we're lonely.

We have a faithful Shepherd when we lose our way.

We have the Commander of the Angel Armies for protection.

It's comforting to know that when I seek Him and ask Him, my Father will meet my needs. As a caregiver to James my needs have changed. I no longer need to hang new curtains in my den, change the color of my dining room walls, redo my guest room every two years, have the most beautiful flowers in the neighborhood, or give the best parties. The things I yearn for now are the things God is already providing for this journey: comfort, courage, endurance, patience, hope, joy, laughter, love, rest, strength, unshakable peace, and wisdom, just to name a few.

In *My Utmost for His Highest, June 9*, Oswald Chambers, that incredibly wise man wrote, "We will have yearnings and desires for certain things...but not until we are at the limit of desperation will we ask... Have you ever asked out of the depths of your total insufficiency and poverty?... A pauper does not ask out of any reason other than the completely hopeless and painful condition of his poverty.... He is not ashamed to beg, 'blessed are the paupers in spirit'" (Matthew 5:3).[55]

Jesus has told us that He has placed a yearning and a longing for perfection in every human heart, something only He can fulfill. Only He is perfect. I yearn for that perfection. I don't want to be mediocre, average, ordinary, complacent or satisfied with the status quo. I want to be completely "sold out" to God. I want to become more like Jesus every day. I yearn to be excellent; to be all God wants me to be. I want to be the best caregiver to James that, with God's help, I can be.

In A.W. Tozer's little book, *The Pursuit of God*, he states: "Complacency is a deadly foe of all spiritual growth. Acute desire must be present, or there will be no manifestation of Christ to His people. He waits to be wanted."[56]

During our homebound years, 2007 through 2010, all my days began at my Bethel. There I was alone with God, equipped with my Bible, a prayer journal, pens and highlighters, and a longing heart. In those days, I was desperate for God. I had such a yearning to find rest from my roller coaster emotions, comfort for my broken heart, strength for my exhausted body, and wisdom for the decisions I faced daily. As I spent time every morning in God's presence, He began to reveal Himself to me in ways I had never before experienced. I had such hunger and thirst for Him, sometimes even an hour was not enough.

---

55   Chambers, *My Utmost for His Highest*, June 9.
56   A.W. Tozer, The Pursuit of God, page 17.

Early one morning, after a troubled night filled with James' restlessness and questions and my strange dreams, I made my way quickly to my Bethel. I prayed, "Father, this morning I am desperate for you." Suddenly I was engulfed in peace so profound I could see it, feel it, and taste it. It was a palpable presence in the room and in my spirit. The presence of God was so real, tears blinded my eyes, and all I could do was praise Him and thank Him. Since that experience, I have had several more "close encounters" with God. I keep them in my Memory Bank for times when I feel fragile or anxious.

The result of a true yearning for God is a yielded life. When we are truly yielded to Him and His will for us, we won't try to attach His name to our "common sense" decisions. We won't lean on our understanding, but we will trust Him in all our ways. When we do this, God will guide us and make our path ahead straight. Everything we once loved and treasured, such as our personal possessions and treasures, our "Stuff," will be secondary to our love for Jesus and our desire for His Lordship over our lives. We will discover that our attachment to and our love of "temporal" things can cause heartache, anxiety, unhappiness, discontentment and ultimate emptiness. I love the old song, "I'd Rather Have Jesus," that says "I'd rather have Jesus than anything this world affords today."

I know personally what it means to let go of "stuff." Many of the things I treasured, things that I thought were so important for my happiness, were sold or given away when we sold our Rainbow Bend house. (I could teach a class: "Downsizing: 101.") Now I realize my things were only temporary and perishable after all. Only the things of God will last.

There is no real joy apart from God. Your situation right now may be almost unbearable:

✝ Your heart may be so heavy you can hardly take a deep breath; you may feel like an elephant is sitting on your chest.

✝ You may feel like you will never be happy or joyful again.

✝ You may long for release from your "prison," the exhaustion and heartache of full-time caregiving.

I understand. I have been there. But I have discovered joy and fulfillment in the Lord, and now that I have tasted His joy, I yearn for more. I have learned that if I take my hunger and my emptiness to Him, He will take His "bucket" of grace and fill my emptiness with everything I need, again and again.

P.S. Beloved, what's on your "Bucket List"? If you haven't already made one, why not do it now? Then lay it unapologetically at God's feet and ask Him to "edit" it according to His perfect will for you. That's one of the things He lovingly does best.

My Prayer — October 19, 2013

"Father, thank You for inspiration and enlightenment as I share with my fellow caregivers the truths You have taught me in our quiet times spent together at my Bethel as I come here daily. I realize that our yearning for more of You has already been fulfilled by Your grace. Even so, sometimes we experience "emptiness" and weariness because of our pursuit of "things" that can never satisfy. Our "stuff," our plans, and many of our passions are dead things. But You, Father, are alive forever. You are my Life, and You have satisfied my thirst, longing, and yearning with a free gift from the spring of the Water of Life (Revelation 21:6).

It is done. Thank You. Father, I will continue to spend the rest of my life loving You." (Lucy)

Plea of a Desperate Caregiver

I am a sad, desperate caregiver, tired and worn,
standing before Your throne, Lord.
I am a ragged traveler, tattered and torn,
with calloused hands and dusty, bleeding feet.
I am drawn to experience Your "presence" by my despair,
and by the depth of my heartache.
I am devastated and humbled
by my relentless neediness.
I am yearning to kneel in Your presence,
just to see Your face.
I know that in Your presence
there is always encouragement for me and grace.
I know I will experience in You what I need
to fill my cup of emptiness.
I know that I will experience in You blessed rest
for my weary body.
I know I will experience in You compassion and comfort
for my loss and loneliness.
I know I will experience in You sweet peace
for my troubled spirit.
I know I will experience in You divine healing
for my wounded, broken heart.
I know that I have nothing to offer You, Lord,
other than my simple, yielded, excepted self.
I know You aways hear and respond to my desperate, earnest plea:
"Lord, because of Your love and mercy, I know You will hold me."
(Lucy)

Zion: Our Real Home

A Deliver stepped down from Zion,
An eternal covenant to make
With the chosen who would love and obey Him;
They're godlessness and sin to take.

There's a huge stone on the road to Zion,
A stone no one can go around.
That stone is Jesus Christ our Savior.
In Him my salvation I found.

I will ask for directions to Zion,
The beautiful city of God
Where I'll finally see sweet Jesus
There on that heavenly sod.

I'm setting my face toward Zion,
Where loved ones and angels wait
In that unshakable, eternal Kingdom
Beyond the pearly gate.

I'm approaching the gates of Zion.
Soon my Father's throne I'll see.
With a grateful heart, I'll praise and worship.
He'll clap His hands and welcome me.

Oh Yes. There's a King in Zion.
A royal banquet awaits me there,
Where on that awesome, Holy Summit
Forever His inheritance I'll share.

~Lucy 2012

God, our Father and Guide, has saved the best for last. This provision, "Zion", our 'real' home, is the last thing we will need. It's our journey's final destination. Only God knows when we will need this provision. Only He knows our departure date. I'm glad the decision is in His hands, not mine. My goal is to live my life in such a way that I am ready at all times to meet my Maker, my Father, my Savior there in Zion, the "beautiful city of God."

My Journal – January 12, 2010

> *"James never feels at home. He constantly says that nothing looks or seems familiar to him anymore. When I ask him what "home" looks like in his mind, he doesn't know. A couple of days ago, we were discussing this. I reminded him that this world is not our home—that we are just passing through on our way to our eternal home in Heaven. I sang a verse of the old familiar song, "This World is not My Home." The words of the song and our discussion gave us hope and a longing for our heavenly home. (Lucy)*

My favorite author, Max Lucado, in one of my favorite daily devotional books, *Grace for the Moment*, wrote, "Unhappiness on earth cultivates a hunger for heaven. By gracing us with a deep dissatisfaction, God holds our attention. We are not happy here because we are not at home here. We are not happy here because we are not supposed to be happy here."[57]

---

57   *Grace for the Moment*, Max Lucado, J. Countryman, a Division of Thomas Nelson, Nashville, Tennessee, 2000.

Although we can always find joy in our relationship with God, this explains our restlessness, our unhappiness. We were not made for the earth as we know it. Thankfully, compared to eternity, our journey through life is brief. When we're enduring hardships, the days and nights may seem endless. But compared to eternity, they are only a "breath." Our days here are given to us to help us learn to think like God, to gain His perspective, and to see things through His eyes. As we begin to see His heart, we become more like Christ, which is His desire and goal for us.

I believe that while we are here our earthly home is very important. There is something "special" about the home. It is a refuge from the stresses and storms of life, a haven for our families and friends. During special occasions like Thanksgiving and Christmas, it becomes a banquet hall, a place for celebrating the joy of being together.

James and I bought our first home a year after we married. It was a new house; we paid $12,000 for it. To me, it was a mansion. I worked very hard to make it comfortable, attractive, warm and welcoming. When our two older boys became teens, we moved to a larger two-story home. In these two homes, during the course of forty-one years, we raised three sons; had countless parties (birthdays and church youth groups), gave wedding and baby showers, housed missionaries on furlough; kept visiting youth evangelists, singing groups, mission groups; kept cancer patients (along with their families) coming here from out of town to M.D. Anderson Hospital for Cancer treatment. Our home became a "haven" for youth who at times, because of dysfunctional family situations, needed a refuge.

Our home has always been a magnet for our sons, their friends and later, their wives, children, and in-laws. There was always room for anyone who needed a place to spend Christmas or Thanksgiving Day.

The last home we bought was our one-story Rainbow Bend "miracle house", the solution to a recommendation by James' Neurologist. She had found evidence of a left frontal lobe stroke he had suffered earlier. Four months later, before we moved into our new home, James was diagnosed with Alzheimer's disease. The ten years we lived in this "perfect house" were some of the happiest and the saddest of our lives. Even with James' advancing illness, we opened our home to family and friends. We had great celebrations. Christmas, Thanksgiving, Easter.

Fourth of July. All with great food, fellowship, and fun. Everyone was always welcome.

As you can see, our home has always been a "special" place. Yours probably has, too. I think in a very small way, this describes Heaven—a place of acceptance, perfect love, indescribable beauty, sweet fellowship, abundance and pure joy. Heaven is a place to praise and serve God, to rest, to lay down our burdens, to celebrate, to be loved forever.

I talk a lot about our Rainbow Bend house—the one "too dear to sell." When, through faith and obedience to God's instructions, I sold that house filled with so many "treasures," my heart was unashamedly broken. Then, in the midst of my sadness, God reminded me that my real "dream house" is in Heaven, already prepared and waiting for me when my journey on earth is ended.

Indulge me for a moment. In my mind's eye, I can see a cozy cottage with a front porch and a swing. The inside is decorated in blue and white; everywhere are bouquets of yellow tulips in cobalt blue vases, and at the windows, white ruffled curtains. The front flowerbeds are filled with my favorite flowers, blue Hydrangeas and blue Plumbago shrubs. There is a heart-shaped wreath on the door with my name on it. When the door is opened, one is greeted by beautiful music and the smell of pumpkin bread, fresh from the oven.

Of course, I'm fantasizing. In my earth-bound mind, I don't know anything about heaven except what the Bible teaches. The one exception that I know of is the amazing account of my dear friend, Don Piper, who died and spent ninety minutes in heaven. He came back and continues to share his experience with thousands of people all over the world, giving hope and encouragement to those whose loved ones have died. Knowing Don, I have absolutely no doubt that everything he shares about his experience is true. It affirms what I already know: that heaven is real and perfect.

In the book of *Revelation*, John, the "disciple Jesus loved," was given a vision of the New Jerusalem coming down out of heaven, the promised place, prepared and ready. John, in *Revelation 21*, did his very best to describe this celestial city in his limited, earthly language.

Many things we won't know about heaven until we get there, but the things I do know make me long for my "real home." The more we know about Heaven, the more "homesick" we will become. While here on earth, we will continue to be "like fish out of water."

My Journal – January 15, 2010

"I was awakened this morning at 4:30. James was praying over and over, "Lord, please, please take me home." I knew that the Lord was also listening because "He never slumbers or sleeps." I lay there for a while, listening until James finally slipped back into a peaceful sleep. Then, I quietly got out of bed, put on my warm robe and slippers and made my way down the hall to my Bethel. I was talking to my Father all the way. I opened His Word and read this wonderful description of Heaven, our final home.

Hebrews 12:22-24: "But you have come to Mount Zion, to the heavenly Jerusalem, the city of the living God. You have come to thousands upon thousands of angels in joyful assembly, to the church of the firstborn, whose names are written in heaven. You have come to God, the judge of all men, to the spirits of righteous men made perfect, to Jesus the mediator of a new covenant, and to the sprinkled blood that speaks a better word than the blood of Abel."

As I read this Scripture, I was reminded that, as God's children, we are travelers passing through this imperfect, hostile world. In First Peter 2:11, we are told that we are "aliens and strangers in the world." Two thousand years after Peter wrote those words, my sweet husband asks me almost every night if he is an "alien." When I tell him "No", he says, "Why then do I feel like an alien? Are you sure I'm not? I don't feel real." This is the same James who has told me every day for the past four years, "I want to go home. I don't

*like it here." I believe that in his dementia, all inhibitions
and all pretense are gone, making him hunger for the real
thing. Heaven.*

*I think that David expressed it perfectly: "I'm asking Yahweh
for one thing, only one thing: to live with him in his house
my whole life long. I'll contemplate his beauty, I'll study at
his feet. That's the only quiet, secure place in a noisy world"
(Psalm 27:4-5 The Message). My prayer for James, my
sweetheart, is that he can feel safe and secure and at peace."
(Lucy)*

My Journal – January 20, 2010

*"Lately, I'm facing so many decisions. It would be so much
easier just to go home to heaven. I've found that it is difficult
to be patient with James when I'm so tired and confused.
I just want to go home to my real home and let my Father
hold me. I long for the things that are waiting for James
and me there: rest, peace, serenity, joy, security. There will be
no more reason to grieve. I can finally lay down my heavy
responsibility of caregiving because James will be well, his
mind healed. We will spend our days praising our faithful
Father.*

*Every sigh, every ache of my heart, every breath I take means
I'm getting closer to home. Every day, as I greet the morning,
I say, "Maybe today, Father. Even so, come quickly Lord
Jesus." I watch the sky for the signs of His return to take us
all home to be with Him in heaven. Until then, I will find
my strength in God to continue to love and care for James.
Also, I will surrender to God's next plans for James and me,
as painful as they may be." (Lucy)*

Have you ever moved into a new house, but it never felt like home? I have. In June of 2011, I had a house built in a beautiful new community around the corner from the Hampton at Pearland, a Brookdale Senior Living Community with an award-winning Memory Care facility, Clare Bridge. James and I had lived there for fourteen months after we sold our "Rainbow Bend" house. I loved the time I spent there. I so needed the rest, and I felt valued and nurtured by everyone. James spent about eight hours each day at Clare Bridge, but I was still caring for him at night. The time came when he simply didn't always feel like getting up early and dressing for breakfast. Many mornings he begged me to let him stay in his recliner and to stay with me, especially when he had not slept the night before. Those mornings, I, too, was often exhausted, and it was easier to keep him with me in our apartment. I would go to the dining room and pick up our breakfast. Some days we even ate our lunch and dinner in our apartment.

I built the house firmly believing that, with full-time help, I could care for James here. The builder converted a small downstairs study near the Master Bedroom into a bedroom with a full bath. It was a perfect "caregiver" space. Also, just in case the time came when I needed to move James full-time back to Clare Bridge, I would be less than a minute away from him. There were several wonderful Care Associates at the Hampton, who were eager to work for me on their days off. They knew and loved James. One young man worked for us for three months. One day he said, "Miss Lucy, there are only so many games of Dominoes you can play in one day." He said, "I think Mr. James is lonely. He needs interaction with his "friends" at Clare Bridge. He needs the mental stimulation he receives there through the "Daily Moments of Success" program."

Of course he did. When I made the agonizing decision to move James back to Clare Bridge full-time, I did it for him, for his happiness and well-being.

A few weeks before my final decision, God confirmed that this was the right thing to do. One evening as we sat in the den, James got out of his recliner and started toward the front door. I said, "Honey, where are you going?" He said, "I'm going home." When I said, "Sit down, you are home," he became agitated and said, "I'm not home, but I'm going home. I wish you would go with me, but if you won't, I still have to go." I finally got him turned around and down the hall to our bedroom, telling him we were going home. I got him ready for bed and crawled in beside him, holding him until he went to sleep. I spent the next hour praying for wisdom and guidance.

A few days later, I received the final answer to my indecision. I was getting James ready for bed. Before getting him into the shower, I took him to the "bathroom." He sat there for a while then said he didn't need to "go." He had been in the shower for a few seconds when he did "go," making a huge "mess." I got him out of the shower and back to the "bathroom" while I cleaned the shower. Then I got him back into the shower, where he immediately made another "mess." When I realized what was happening, I yelled "No" at the top of my voice. By the time I got James and the shower cleaned up again, and got him to bed, I was "frazzled" to put it mildly. Still smelling of disinfectant, I climbed gratefully into bed. At exactly two o'clock, James woke me. He said, "Lucy. Lucy. I have something very important to tell you." I said, "James, it's the middle of the night. Can't it wait until morning?" He said, "No. I have to tell you now. You've got to stop abusing me." I said "Honey, I would never abuse you." He said, "Yes, you do, and you have to stop abusing me." I knew at that moment that my decision was made.

It was the right decision, even though it broke my heart. From the very first day, October 1, 2011, James "blossomed" with all the attention and activity. But when I returned to our house without him, it was just a house, never a home. I realized that no place where I would live here on earth would ever again feel like home without James. When James died from heart failure and pneumonia on September 17, 2012, I watched as he was gloriously and immediately transported to his "real home," heaven. As he took his last breaths, I whispered in his ear, "James, you're going to see Jesus, and I'm a little envious because you're going to see Him first." I could imagine him looking into the face of Jesus, and Jesus saying, "Welcome home, James. You are at your real home here with Me, forever."

I want you to remember that, when life gets difficult, we're just passing through this imperfect world. The path on our long weary journey as caregivers is filled with heartaches and discouragement. That is why God packed so many wonderful provisions for our journey—everything we would need—from A to Z, from Angels to Zion!

Although, as caregivers, we encounter landslides and roadblocks, potholes and detours, bends in the road, oceans of tears, desert wildernesses of emptiness, and valleys of sorrow, this long road will finally lead us home. When we think about that beautiful place that Jesus has prepared for those of us who have given our hearts to Him for His dwelling place, we will find the courage for the rest of the journey.

In the meantime, I plan to celebrate each day, savoring the beauty and blessings of life. I will be spending time with God in the "secret place" where I will continue to find peace and joy and boundless love. At my Bethel, I will open His Word daily to find the wisdom I need for each day. There God will continue to reveal His plans and purpose for the next season of my journey, "Life after Caregiving."

Chapter 13

The Last Mile

My Journal – August 29, 2012

"Today when I went to Clare Bridge at noon to have lunch with James, I found him sitting in the living room instead of in the dining room. He refused to get out of the chair where he was sitting, even to move to the love seat we usually shared. When I brought a tray containing his lunch, he refused to eat, even when I offered to feed him. When I asked if he felt bad, he said, "Yes. Can I go?" I assured him that God would decide exactly the right time, and I walked him back to his room, to his recliner. I sat with him until he went to sleep, then I slipped away. I sensed that this was a "shadow" of things to come." (Lucy)

My Journal – August 30, 2012

"I arrived at Clare Bridge at 11:55, just as lunch was being served. James was not at his table. I found him sitting in an armchair in the hall outside his room. He said, "I can't go any further. Can I just sleep?" He refused lunch. I did get him to drink a little Ensure. Then I walked him across the hall back into his room for a nap. The "shadow" remains. (Lucy)

My Journal – September 5, 2012

"Today is James' eighty-sixth birthday. I went to my local grocery store this morning and purchased a helium balloon with the words, "Happy Birthday to my Hero." I also bought enough miniature chocolate cupcakes with "decadent chocolate frosting" and colorful sprinkles for all the residents and associates at Clare Bridge. When I arrived, everyone was in the dining room. I thought James would be delighted with the balloon as I tied it to his chair, but he was quiet, not his usual funny, happy self. When he refused to eat a chocolate cupcake, I knew he was not himself. The "shadow" is growing larger. (Lucy)

My Journal – September 8, 2012

"Today is Saturday. I was up at my usual 6:30 A.M. What was not usual was that I had dressed and put on makeup after having my coffee and my "quiet time" with God. My plan was to visit James at Clare Bridge this morning to encourage him to eat breakfast, something he had not been doing for the past week. At 8:30, as I picked up my keys and purse, my cell phone rang. When I answered, I heard these words, "Miss Lucy, we're calling "911" for Mr. James." Without asking "Why?" I said, "Don't call. I'll be there in 30 seconds (which I was)." On the way, I was thanking God for the house He had led me to build around the corner from Clare Bridge. When I arrived, James was sitting on

"our love seat," surrounded by several Care Associates. He was "laboriously" breathing and appeared very pale. One associate explained that he had suddenly become short of breath and complained of dizziness. Another brought his wheel chair (which he never used) and helped me get him into my car. Within ten minutes from the time I had received the phone call, I was at the entrance to Memorial Herman Hospital ER.

An emergency room attendant came out immediately with a wheelchair and took James inside while I parked the car. Everyone in the ER was wonderful. They quickly admitted James, who, by now, was making every effort to be his usual charming self.

The next few hours were filled with the normal tests, EKG, Chest X-Ray, lab work, breathing treatment, monitoring of O_2 levels, and observation by various nurses and ER doctors. After the breathing treatment, James felt better and was again being his sweet, funny self, charming everyone who came to his ER room. By now, our son David, had come and was joking with his Dad, as usual.

Finally, a young ER doctor came and explained that James was being admitted to the hospital overnight for heart monitoring and several other tests, including a Nuclear Heart Scan and an Echo-cardiogram. He reported that the chest x-ray did not show any pneumonia, which is always a danger for elderly Alzheimer's patients. (Lucy)

My Journal – September 9, 2012

By 1:00 P.M. yesterday, James and I were settled in a private room with a window-seat couch. James slept off and on, waking only when a nurse came to replace the electrodes that he frequently removed from his chest, forgetting of course why they were there. David had gone home and our son, Matt, had come to stay with his Dad while I ran home to get a change of clothes and some personal care items (I didn't need these, after all). Alzheimer's patients must have someone, a family member or friend, with them at all times. When I returned to the hospital just before dusk, I learned that Matt had gone with his Dad to Radiology where James was having a Nuclear Heart Scan. I relieved Matt, who was exhausted physically and emotionally from assisting the technician in keeping James still and calm.

Later, back in his room, James ate one bite of his dinner, and I ate the rest. (We had both missed breakfast and lunch.) Now began the long, long night. I stood by the bed all night to keep James from climbing over the side rails of his bed. He had an I.V. in one arm and an indwelling urinary catheter. Every time James put his leg over the short side rail, a loud buzzer sounded, and a nurse came running. This went on all night. Because James was scheduled for an echo-cardiogram the next morning, sedation was not an option. Neither were restraints. Just me. I often looked longingly at the small couch nearby, needing desperately to lay down my weary head and to stretch out my tired back and legs. But that was not possible. Several times, I became impatient with James and tried in vain to explain to him why he could not get up—something I later regretted. James was adamant. He was "going home to his 'real' home."

Thankfully, this morning finally arrived with more blood tests and monitoring of blood pressure and O_2 levels. James refused to eat any of his breakfast. At this point, he had not eaten any food for at least thirty-six hours and had drunk only enough water to take his medications. No one except me seemed to be concerned about this. It was late morning when a technician came to do an Echo-cardiogram that would produce an image of James' heart. We were told that the cardiologist on call that weekend would come in later to give us the results.

It took me back to Saturday in March of 1994. James experienced some chest pain while mowing the grass. I called our doctor who saw him in his office as soon as we could get there. His diagnosis was "angina" (I already suspected that.) He gave James a prescription for Niacin and ordered him to rest until we could see a cardiologist on Monday. The cardiologist was Dr. Bapat, whose office was next to Memorial Herman S.E. Hospital. He saw James on Monday morning and, after examining him, he scheduled a heart catheterization for that afternoon. When he discovered several blockages, he had James taken that evening by ambulance to St. Lukes Hospital in the Houston Medical Center. This amazing doctor had arranged for James to have quadruple coronary artery bypass surgery early the next morning, no doubt preventing a major heart attack.

Before you start snoring, I am going somewhere with this story. Early afternoon, while I was still standing by James' bed, trying to keep him calm, the cardiologist on call came into the room. Are you ready for this? It was Dr. Bapat, our dear friend whom we had not seen for at least ten years. I don't know who was more surprised. I said, "It's you." And he said, "And it's you." I think we both knew that this was no coincidence. While a nurse stayed with James, Dr. Bapat took me to the nurses' station and showed me the images of James' heart. He said, "Lucy, the warranty on James' coronary artery bypass has expired. His heart is completely worn out." He told me that I should call in hospice for James and contact our internist's office to arrange this.

When we went back into the room, James said, "You're too wonderful to be real. Can I go home? I want to go to my real home." Dr. Bapat took James' hand and said, "James, dear friend, you are going home to your "real home" very soon." He knew what James meant, and he knew, without a doubt where James was going. As he was leaving, we shook hands, and he said that he didn't know how long it would be, but that it would be soon.

Matt came to the hospital to help me get his Dad back to Clare Bridge, and I shared with him what Dr. Bapat had said. James was exhausted and as soon as we arrived at Clare Bridge, one of the associates brought his wheelchair and took him to his room to get him ready for bed.

I was also exhausted, but I needed to take Matt back to the hospital to pick up his truck. Then I made the difficult calls to David and Tim. The news was bittersweet. It was something we had all prayed for, yet had dreaded. Then I called our doctor who made all the arrangements for Hallmark Hospice to take over James' care, starting tomorrow." (Lucy)

My Journal Entry – Monday, September 10, 2012

"As of 1:30 P.M. yesterday, James and I are traveling the final mile of our journey. Yesterday, our dear friend and cardiologist, Dr. Bapat, gave us the itinerary for the rest of the journey. We have now entered our last season together—the 'Hospice Season'. Some of the Hallmark Hospice personnel met me at Clare Bridge today to discuss what we could expect during this 'season'. They also delivered a hospital bed and many supplies to James' room. I already know and love Laura, the R.N. I've always told her that when we reached this time, I wanted her to care for James. Hospice will be a great comfort to me and relief for the loving Care Associates here at Clare Bridge. With all their support, I feel like a "warm blanket" is covering me.

Our son, Tim, called from San Antonio to tell me that he, Kathy and Jacob are coming this weekend. We are planning for the whole family to be together at Clare Bridge on Saturday to take pictures with James and to spend time with him while he is still able to enjoy it. There is a strange sense of urgency. I know that God is working out the details for these days. And I will be spending all of my time with James." (Lucy)

My Journal – September 15, 2012

"This has been a memorable day. Tim and his family came this morning. In the afternoon, our entire family gathered at Clare Bridge. James sat on 'our love seat' in the Common Area while everyone gathered around him for pictures and hugs. James was loving every minute of all this attention. I could tell that he was very tired, and occasionally he dozed off for a second. Then he was joking and teasing and grinning like old times. Matt was there with Matthew and Micah. David and Pam were there with Adam and Brett. Tim and Kathy were there with Jacob. I looked at our eight wonderful boys, looking so much like their "handsome" Dad and Papaw, and I was so grateful for the legacy James would be leaving them. I realized again how much God has blessed our family and how blessed I am to be James' wife and the mother and grandmother of his sons and grandsons. "Father, thank you for this special time You have given us. I know it will be very hard for Tim and his family to leave tonight, knowing that this could be the last time they will spend with James. Comfort them and keep them safe." (Lucy)

My Journal – September 16, 2012

"Matt and I stopped by Clare Bridge on our way to church this morning. Laura was here checking on James. The hospice aide had given him a bath this morning, dressed him, and brushed his hair. He looked so fresh and sweet. I noticed

that his nail beds were bluish, and his skin had a strange pallor. Laura said that his vital signs were good, and his breathing was about the same. They were going to get him up to sit in his wheelchair for a while. After church, Matt and I picked up ice cream for James, thinking he might enjoy it, but he refused it. Dr. Bapat had told us last week that it was perfectly normal to not want to eat when death was near, and that I should not worry about his refusal to eat or drink anything. The nurse was getting ready to put James to bed for a nap, so I kissed him and promised to be back before he woke up. Then I went home to change clothes. It was a 'surreal' time. I remembered that, when my mother was dying, I had gone to get my hair and nails done. As I sat in the salon, surrounded by people having normal conversations, normal activities, normal lives, I felt strangely out of place as if I were dreaming. Now, as I got out of my car, some neighbors waved; some were mowing their lawn; others were walking their dogs. I wanted to shout, "Don't you know that my sweetheart is dying?"

I changed clothes, rested for a while, called David and Tim to report on their Dad, and then drove back the short distance to Clare Bridge. James was sitting in his recliner with his eyes closed but when I said, "James, your beautiful wife is here," he opened his eyes and grinned. I pulled a chair close to him and held his hands. They were cold, and I noticed that the palms were purplish in color. As I held those dear, familiar hands, I thought about the fact that soon they would hold the hand of God. This was a special, sacred time that I wanted to preserve and keep stored in my memory forever. As the sun went down, Laura came. I had planned to spend the night, but she encouraged me to go home and get a good night's sleep. She said that James was stable and that an aide would be with him all during the night. So I came home to try to sleep. When I'm not sleeping, I will be praying. (Lucy)

❦

Monday, September 17, 2012, 10:00 P.M.

"This will be the hardest, most painful journaling I will ever do, but I must do it. The story of our journey would not be complete without it. I was up very early. I spent a few minutes at my "Bethel," asking God to cover us with His peace. Then I dressed quickly and drove to Clare Bridge. Before I could ring the doorbell, one of my favorite Care Associates opened the door. She said, "Miss Lucy, something's wrong with Mr. James. We had trouble waking him up, and he can't talk." They had already called Laura from hospice, and she was standing by his bed when I went in. James' eyes were closed, and he was breathing heavily and irregularly. I went to him and bent over and began to talk to him. He tried to open his eyes, and he mumbled something I couldn't understand. I kissed him then stepped out into the hall to call David and Matt, who were at work. I went back to stand by James, leaning down so that he could hear what I wanted to tell him: "James, it's Lucy. I love you so much, but it's getting close to the time for you to go to your "real home." I know that's where you want to be. It's okay for you to go. Jesus is waiting for you. I'll be alright because Jesus will be with me, too."

All this time, Laura had been working with James, elevating his head to help him breath. I think she and I were both surprised that the end was coming so quickly, and she was trying to make him as comfortable as possible. By now David had come and was standing by his Dad. I made another quick call to Matt to be sure he was on his way. David had called Pam earlier, and she was on her way.

James' breathing was now very labored and irregular. Laura lowered his head a little, and she and I turned him onto his right side. She asked me about giving him morphine to relax him. I felt that we should try to wait for Matt and Pam, but I wanted James to be as comfortable as possible, so I said, "Yes, if it will help." Then I again leaned over very close and said these words into James' left ear, "James, you're getting ready to see Jesus. I'm a little jealous because you are going to see Him first. Wait for me; I'll be there soon."

As soon as I finished speaking, James took one last breath, then was still. His journey was over. He was with Jesus. There had been no pain, no suffering. David and I (and Laura) were "in shock." As I leaned over and put my head on James' chest, I saw Pam come in. She and David held one another and cried. Then Matt was beside me. When he realized that his Dad was gone, and he had not been there, I could tell that his heart was breaking.

My heart was breaking for my children, but I was engulfed in peace that was so profound, it was like a Presence in the room. Laura was busy making calls to her office who would notify the Hospice Chaplain, the Coroner, and Mr. Niday at Niday Funeral Home, with whom we had made funeral plans several years ago.

Then I made the very difficult call to our son, Tim, who had been here with James on Saturday. I told him that his Dad had died so peacefully, so gently, so painlessly—the gift of a loving Father to a faithful son. Tim was devastated but thankful, as we all were, that his Dad had not suffered and that he was with God.

Word of James' death had spread quickly through Clare Bridge and into the whole Hampton Community. Within a few minutes, groups of employees began to gather outside James' room. Most of them were sobbing; some were openly weeping. Then two or three at a time came in to see "Mr. James" one last time. They hugged me and cried, many of them sharing how much James' love and humor had touched *and enriched their lives. They all came: Administrators, office staff, nursing staff, care associates from every building, maintenance, housekeeping and kitchen staff. As they came, I comforted them, and they comforted me with the stories they shared about James and the love they felt for him.*

The Niday Funeral Home personnel had come, but they patiently and respectfully waited until the last person had visited James' room. The last one to come was one of the cooks who had come twice before, and she apologized to me: "I'm so sorry, Miss Lucy, but I had to see Mr. James just one more time. He's the only person who has ever made me feel special or beautiful. I'll miss him so much." I hugged her and told her that I would never forget her.

Matt, David, Pam, and I were so touched by this amazing display of love and grief for the one we all loved so much. We waited together in the Common Area at Clare Bridge until the funeral home personnel took James, then we stood with the Hospice Chaplain as he prayed a beautiful, comforting prayer. We all left there in our cars to go to my house to make some calls and to process what had happened. We were all still in shock from the suddenness of James' death. After all, it had only been eight days since Dr. Bapat had given us the news about James' heart. I guess we were all thinking weeks instead of days. But we had no regrets, only gratitude. I think I will sleep well tonight, knowing that James is finally Home." (Lucy)

Tim, Kathy and Jacob came on Wednesday. Together we all planned, with God's help, a beautiful funeral that would honor James and bring glory to God. The funeral would be at our church on Saturday morning. On Friday evening, the Niday Funeral Home Chapel was filled to overflowing several times for over two hours. People came from everywhere—our sons' friends and co-workers; friends from the three churches where James and I had served for over 50 years. Our son Matt's church, Grace, had ministered faithfully to James and me after we moved to the Hampton, and many of our friends and several of the church staff from there came. Friends of Tim and Kathy came from San Antonio. Our neighbors, old and new came. The most surprising visitor was James' former boss, the District Manager of Lubricant Sales for Shell Oil Company. I had called to inform him of James' death, and he said he would be at the Funeral Home, and he was. He shook our sons' hands and held mine as he shared with us how very special James was and what a great contribution he made, personally and professionally, to Shell Oil Company the forty years he was there.

There was so much love in that room all evening that I felt like I was being carried on eagle's wings. I was "high" on love and grace. After the personnel at Niday had gently but firmly escorted the last lingering guest to the exit, they shared that in all their years, they had never seen such an outpouring of love and respect. I thought about how humbled James would have been by so much attention. I was certainly amazed and humbled by all the love poured out on our family.

The funeral on Saturday was all that I could have wished for and more. It honored James' life and brought glory to the Lord he loved so much. The church was packed with people from all over the city and state. As soon as the service was over, Mr. Niday himself drove the hearse to Bedias, Texas where James and I have cemetery lots and a headstone already in place. As he quickly moved the casket, our family stayed and visited with guests in the church foyer.

After a beautiful luncheon prepared and served by the Children's Ministry, we left the church and drove to the cemetery in Bedias for a sweet graveside service followed by a meal prepared and served by members at Bedias Baptist Church. It is the church James' family has belonged to since the 19th century. It is the church where James asked Jesus into his twelve-year-old heart during Vacation Bible School.

After the meal we all returned to our homes. It was dark by the time I arrived home, and I was very tired. I gratefully removed my not-so-comfortable dress shoes in which I had walked many miles in the last twelve hours. I dressed for bed, then walked out on the back deck and looked up at the star-studded sky. Suddenly, a shooting star made a bright arc across the night sky, then it was gone. At that moment, I felt a powerful sense of God's presence with me. I wish I could find the words to tell you exactly how I felt. I wanted to climb onto the roof and tell the whole world that we have a Father in Heaven who loves us so much that He would take the time to deliver to me such a beautiful love message, just when I needed it most. I knew He had done it for me on this night that I had dreaded since I fell in love with James fifty-six years ago, this month. I stood there for a minute more, thanking and praising God. Then I came inside. As I turned down the covers to climb into bed, I remembered a small, blue velvet bag Jack Niday had given me at the cemetery. I found it in my purse and removed from it James' lapel pin with the four diamonds' which represent his forty years with Shell Oil Company. Then I removed his wedding band that I had placed on his finger on November 9, 1957. I slipped it on the middle finger of my right hand. It fit perfectly. As I got into bed, Satan tried to tell me that James was all alone in that dark, lonely cemetery in Bedias. Then Jesus told me, in my spirit, "Lucy, James is here with me. You and James have finished the last mile of your thirteen-year journey with Alzheimer's and you finished well."

Then I touched James' ring and went to sleep.

The Last Mile Together

So many times on this journey, I have asked God "How long,
Lord?" The "how" and "why" questions came without warning,
followed by His Words, "Trust Me", and we did,
James and I.

When the answer came one day, I was sad, but at peace.
I knew that the rapid failure of his beautiful heart would
soon take my sweetheart to his "real" home, free
of Alzheimer's. Now we walk the last mile together,
James and I.

As our days together ticked steadily away, we spent some time
in the beautiful garden at Clare Bridge where James now lived,
always happiest and at peace when we were together,
James and I.

Late one evening we sat watching the sunset, marveling at the
breathtaking colors transforming the western horizon, holding each
other's dear familiar hand, lovingly sharing our "sunset time" together,
James and I.

As we sat close together on the small garden bench, I tried not to think
of the inevitable approaching loss and emptiness ahead, trying
instead to focus on our precious togetherness,
James and I.

Often, on the last two days, as we snuggled on
our "love seat" at Clare Bridge,
the same questions were asked again and again, the
same answers lovingly and patiently given as we sat together,
James and I.

The last day we sat together, no words were spoken; none were needed.
Our hearts were overflowing with what we had
always felt and known;
we shared silently a love that thirteen years
of Alzheimer's could not diminish,
James and I.

Finally, nothing mattered but the love between us that had
grown so deep we finally shared one heart; the knowledge
that our journey was ending made these sacred moments
more precious, just being together,
James and I.

The last evening, as I held him close, our love silent but immeasurably deep, I wondered how I could live in the world without him, loving him desperately as we sat quietly together, James and I.

When there was nothing I could do to hold back the night, I kissed his dear mouth for the last time. As I helped tuck him into bed, I quoted his familiar bedtime pledge, till death do us part," still together for now, James and I.

Then came the morning. James was somewhere between here and his "real home." There was nothing I could do to stop the ticking clock. Hours became minutes; minutes, seconds – then stillness. James is with Jesus. But I am not alone. We grieve and celebrate together, God and I.

~ *Lucy*

(Inspired by a poem by Paul Marian: "When We Walked Together," from Deaths and Transfigurations. (Paraclete Press, 2005)

Chapter 14

Reflections

"In this you greatly rejoice, though now
for a little while, you may have had to suffer grief
in all kinds of trials. These have come so that
your faith – of greater worth than gold, which
perishes even though refined by fire – may be
proved genuine and may result in praise, glory and
honor when Jesus Christ is revealed"
(1 Peter 1:6-7)

In this life, there are all kinds of suffering and grief, all kinds of trials. Mine can't compare with those of women like Elisabeth Elliot or Gracia Burnham, missionaries who lost their godly husbands at the hands of brutal men. As I read their stories of their trials, I am humbled to be counted as a woman who has suffered grief and trials on my journey with James, my godly husband. Our enemy was not brutal men. It was the brutal enemy Alzheimer's disease which, for thirteen years, ruthlessly robbed my husband of his memory, his logic, his reasoning, and his mind.

Those years of grief and trials, however, were not wasted. Although we were forced to rethink our priorities, one priority never changed. We were committed to living our lives in a way that would continue to bring honor and glory to God and love and encouragement to everyone we met along the way. We would continue to serve God with every opportunity we were given. God honored our commitment by giving James, even in his dementia, many opportunities to bring love, joy and laughter to everyone, wherever he went. Even at Clare Bridge, he spread so much love, "blooming faithfully where he was planted." The

Spirit of God that lived in his heart never got dementia, and it shone brightly until God took him home.

God gave me supernatural health, strength and energy to care for James. He gave me unshakable peace and joy in the midst of heartache and loneliness. Most importantly, He gave me a stronger, more genuine faith to trust Him and to be a testimony to others of His faithfulness in the midst of adversity.

With God's guidance, I learned to stay on the path He had planned instead of wandering off into the past or the future. I learned to stay focused on the moment because that's all we had. Actually, for James the "moment" was everything. I learned to trust God completely with my circumstances, knowing and believing that He had planned my destiny before I was born. "Like an open book, you watched me grow from conception to birth; all the stages of my life all prepared before I'd even lived one day" (Psalm 139:16 *The Message*)

As I said earlier in the book, I believe that God placed James and me on this journey with Alzheimer's for such a time as this "to be a light in the growing darkness of dementia." Those who are caught in the darkness of this frightening epidemic that is Alzheimer's disease will need the stories of the "Pioneers" who have traveled the difficult road of Alzheimer's and have successfully reached their destination—stronger, wiser, and victorious. It was this belief that I clung to every day for thirteen years as I sought God's directions and instructions. I constantly prayed for His guidance and wisdom. In answer to my prayers, God became our faithful Guide.

As the years passed, God's boundless love carried me through many dark valleys; across dry, lonely deserts; over treacherous mountain passes. It protected me through dangerous storms and held me close during thousands of dark, sleepless nights. It gave me guidance and direction when I got off the trail and temporarily lost my way. God's love always found me. I was never out of His sight; to Him, I was never lost.

To be completely honest, there were times I wanted to give up, to tell God, "stop this journey, I want to get off." Sometimes when the road was dark and rough, I would say with the psalmist, "How long, O Lord? How long?" (Psalm 89:46). I would say, "Father, how long must James and I endure this tragedy of Alzheimer's?"

God could have given me a date. I know that. But instead, He gave me endurance and patience, strength and courage, comfort and hope, and miraculous health. He gave me a daily invitation to walk with Him, to roll my burdens onto His shoulders. He who lives forever and who is the same yesterday, today, and forever never left my side. He reminded me in His Word that this journey is brief compared to an eternity spent with Him in heaven; that it will be worth it all when I see Jesus.

On September 17, 2012, our journey with Alzheimer's ended. God, the Source of all power, gently and compassionately unplugged the earthly cord to James' beautiful heart and took him to Heaven, his "Real Home." God was there with me that day to wrap me in His love and peace as I experienced the bittersweet ending of our long journey.

Yes, James and I have been on a very long journey. Looking back, I realize that, like any journey, there were wonderful, memorable experiences; there were some not so wonderful. There were beautiful sunny days; there were dark, stormy days. There were wide, smooth highways; there were rough, difficult trails.

James and I traveled every mile, the easy and the difficult, with an awareness of God's presence. The smooth highways were clearly His blessings. But the rough trails? Those He used to drive us to our knees to prepare us and give us strength for what lay ahead.

The greatest blessing was knowing that we had the best Guide one could ask for. He provided everything we needed for our long journey. By His grace, He provided a special blessing, the means for James to spend the last year of his life in Clare Bridge, Brookdale's highly rated community for Alzheimer's and Dementia Care. This wonderful facility, thirty seconds away from my house, provided a secure and happy environment for James. As I visited him there several times a day, I was always amazed by their Daily Moments of Success program which is deeply rooted in the philosophy of Person Centered Care and which gives purpose and meaning to the lives of the residents. James was obviously very well cared for, and he was obviously happy. He loved all the attention he received from the Care Associates and the many visitors. I loved the fact that I was free to love and enjoy him, to spend quality time with him without the stress and exhaustion of twenty-four hour days as his full-time Caregiver. We snuggled together on our special love seat; we walked in the beautiful garden together. We laughed and sometimes danced during the wonderful parties there. James often said, "I love it when you come to my parties."

One of God's sweetest gifts to me was James Dishongh, the perfect traveling companion in sickness and health. Even in his dementia, he was:

♥ Cheerful, loving, and funny. "I love you more than you'll ever know." "Have you always been that pretty?" "You're too wonderful to be real."

♥ Considerate. "Are you okay? Are you sure?"

♥ Easy going and uncomplaining. "I'm doing great." "I'm just fine."

♥ Encouraging and tolerant. "It'll be okay." "Don't worry."

♥ Helpful. "Can I help you?" "I'm not an invalid. What is an invalid anyway?"

♥ Honest to a fault. "I can't eat a cookie from this package. We haven't paid for it yet." (Spoken at Randall's while we were shopping one day)."

♥ Content and steady as a rock. "We're so blessed. Why are we so blessed?" "I love it here."

Shortly after James' death, after all the necessary paper work was finished and everyone who needed to know had been notified, I took a deep breath and took stock of the future. A future without Alzheimer's.

A future without James.

On October 3, 2012, I packed a bag and took my tired body and my bruised heart to San Antonio, Texas, to spend time with Tim and his family. I hadn't had an opportunity to spend time with them in their lovely home because I had not wanted to leave James, even for a day, to go that far away. The guest room in their home is decorated in my favorite colors, blue and white. It is a quiet, soothing room where I could spend time resting and recovering from my long, exhausting journey.

On Friday morning, October 5, 2012, I had the great privilege of being at my grandson's school for Grandparent's Day. That was my main objective for being at my son's at this particular time. After a special Grammar School Assembly, I visited my grandson's classroom where I met his teacher and watched as he and his classmates presented a sweet program for their grandparents. I met his friends; then he presented me with a gift he had made. Afterward, we had lunch together in a special place set up just for students and their grandparents. It was so much fun. In my heart, I kept thanking God for all this unexpected joy at a time when I needed it most. I couldn't help thinking how much James would have loved all of this.

After lunch, my son picked me up at the school. We spent some quality time together, just the two of us, talking as we strolled through downtown Boerne, stopping occasionally to go into one of the interesting shops along the way. I love, love, love Boerne, a quaint, picturesque town in the beautiful Texas Hill Country.

After school, we met my daughter-in-law, her mother, and my grandson, at a historical hotel in Boerne where we had dinner in an elegant dining room. I kept pinching myself to be sure I wasn't just dreaming this. As the sun began to set, we returned home.

At the end of this "perfect day," I went to bed in my blue and white "haven of rest," exhausted but completely relaxed and content. I slept like a baby for the first time in a long time. At 6:00 A.M. I suddenly awoke, aware that I had experienced something extraordinary. I had dreamed that James and I were at Hermann Park in Houston, Texas. We were sitting on a small bench near the stage at Miller Outdoor Theater. We often took our sons there when they were children.

I said to James, "Honey, I'm going up on the stage to sing. I want you to promise you will stay right here. Don't move from this bench." James said, "Okay, I promise." When I reached the stage and took the mike, I turned around. James was gone. I panicked, but it was too late. The music had started – only it wasn't my music. It was the most beautiful music I had ever heard. I realized that the audience had turned to look to my right. Then I saw James, sitting on the stage to my right, playing a harp. Spellbound, I stood until the beautiful song was finished. James then got up, walked over to me, took my hand and we stepped off the stage together. As we walked, I looked down at James' feet. I said, "James, you're getting mud on your favorite sandals." And he said, "I don't need them anymore."

I slid out of bed and onto my knees, acutely aware of God's presence. I knew that for the second time since James' death, God had sent me a message that James is with Him, alive and well (Not that I ever doubted it).

This dream was, and still is, one of the most profound experiences in my entire life. It was several days before I could share this dream with anyone. I wanted to keep it for myself, to savor it and to hold it in my heart—this sacred gift from my heavenly Father. The dream was so symbolic, especially the "harp" and the beautiful music. I wasn't sure that anyone would believe me, much less realize the significance of it.

For me, this experience was the perfect ending to the story of a beautiful life and a beautiful love between two people, love that was not changed or diminished by Alzheimer's disease. Our love was a constant, giving meaning and purpose to our fifty-five years together. Our love lives on even though death has taken James home.

I still miss him every day. He smiles at me from his picture that I keep by my bed. Sometimes God reminds me: "Lucy, James was my gift to you while he was there on earth, but he was never yours to keep. His life began with Me. He had a wonderful life filled with the love and joy you gave him. Now, after eighty-six years, he is again with me. We are waiting for you here in your "real home." I know the time, so you needn't worry about when. Just trust Me and realize that life is a gift from Me. Enjoy it and treasure every moment until you join us here. In the meantime, continue to fill your life with all the things I have planned for your new journey, your new normal—life after Alzheimer's."

Beloved fellow caregiver, as I write the last few words of our story, I'm already missing the time I've spent thinking of you. Maybe we'll meet in person one day soon. I hope so.

In closing, there are five things I want you to remember as you walk your journey with Alzheimer's:

1. Never give up. "Don't quit. Don't cave in. It is all well worth it in the end." (Matthew 10:22 *The Message*).

2. On the days when life gives you lemons, ask God to help you make the most amazing, unforgettable, delicious lemonade the world has ever tasted.

3. Love unconditionally with everything in you, even when it hurts. Mark Twain said it best: "Love like you've never been hurt.[58]

4. God loves you with a never-ending love, and He will be walking with you until the end of your journey.

5. Always be courageous, knowing that caregiving really is a "high calling!"

---

58   On a bookmark by Driftwood Design.